The People's Guide to Vitamins and Minerals

The People's Guide to Vitamins and Minerals

from A to Zinc

Dominick Bosco

CONTEMPORARY
BOOKS, INC.
CHICAGO

Library of Congress Cataloging in Publication Data

Bosco, Dominick.
    The people's guide to vitamins and minerals,
from A to Zinc.

    Includes bibliographical references and index.
    1. Vitamins.   2. Minerals in the body.
I. Title.
QP771.B66   1980   613.2'8   79-8743
ISBN 0-8092-7140-0
ISBN 0-8092-7139-7 pbk.

Published by Contemporary Books, Inc.
180 North Michigan Avenue, Chicago, Illinois 60601
Manufactured in the United States of America
Library of Congress Catalog Card Number: 79-8743
International Standard Book Number: 0-8092-7140-0 (cloth)
                                    0-8092-7139-7 (paper)

Published simultaneously in Canada by
Beaverbooks, Ltd.
150 Lesmill Road
Don Mills, Ontario M3B 2T5
Canada

Contents

introduction : Can Vitamins Make You Healthier?   1

section 1 : VITAMINS   17

  1 : Vitamin A   *19*

  2 : Thiamine (B_1)   *34*

  3 : Riboflavin (B_2)   *44*

  4 : Niacin (B_3)   *51*

  5 : Pyridoxine (B_6)   *61*

  6 : Folate   *78*

  7 : Cobalamin (B_{12})   *91*

  8 : Biotin   *100*

  9 : Pantothenate (Pantothenic Acid)   *105*

10 : Choline   *114*

11 : Inositol   *120*

12 : PABA   *122*

13 : Vitamin C   *125*

14 : Vitamin D   *155*

15 : Vitamin E   *163*

16 : Vitamin K   *184*

section 2 : MINERALS   **187**

17 : Calcium   189
18 : Chromium   201
19 : Copper   209
20 : Fluorine   212
21 : Iodine   218
22 : Iron   221
23 : Magnesium   227
24 : Manganese   234
25 : Molybdenum   237
26 : Phosphorus   238
27 : Potassium   241
28 : Selenium   245
29 : Silicon   251
30 : Sodium   255
31 : Zinc   257
32 : Other Minerals   269

section 3 : PARTNERS, OUTLAWS,
            AND QUESTIONS   **271**

33 : Bioflavonoids   273
34 : The Outlaw Vitamins   278
35 : The Eight Most Asked Questions   285
    Notes   293
    Index   315

Introduction

Can Vitamins Make You Healthier?

At the heart of everyone's curiosity about vitamins is the question *What can vitamins do for me?* People want to know what vitamins and minerals are capable of and what they're not. They want to know exactly how important vitamins and minerals are in life, whether or not they can look to vitamins and minerals as a means to improve health, whether they should be taking more of them, which ones they should be taking, and whether it's dangerous to take "too much" of them.

Here's one way to address those questions: *If any one or more of the vitamins or minerals in this book were completely removed from your diet for a long enough time, you would become miserably ill and eventually die.* With some of the vitamins or minerals, death might not occur for many months or even years. With others, it would come in a matter of weeks.

Such an absolute deficiency of any vitamin or mineral is

1

practically impossible, of course, except in a laboratory. But we're not really concerned with deficiencies so severe. We assume our diets are providing all the vitamins and minerals.

What we want to know is *What can MORE vitamins and minerals in my diet do for me?* Can we improve upon good health?

Let's approach the question this way: There is a continuum between severe illness and optimum health. We're all *somewhere* on that continuum, and we all want to move toward optimum health and away from illness. Can vitamins and minerals help us do that?

Yes.

Even if we're already getting enough of them in our diet?

The only way to answer that question is to begin with another question: How do you *know* you're getting enough vitamins and minerals in your diet? What is "enough"?

Say you're at a certain point on that continuum and you're satisfied with your general health, your performance at work and play, and your relations with other people. But you buy a few dollars' worth of vitamin and mineral supplements and start taking them, anyway. A couple of months later you suddenly realize you haven't had a cold for a long time; that ache in your shoulder is gone; your gums don't bleed when you brush your teeth; you don't get sleepy in the middle of the afternoon anymore; you're getting more and better work done; your tennis has improved; you feel better about yourself; and you're getting along better with your family and friends.

You've moved closer to the optimum health end of the continuum, and it appears the vitamins and minerals have helped you do it. Now that you're getting more vitamins and minerals in your diet, you're *better* than you were before. Obviously, the amounts you were getting before weren't "enough."

Another example: Two people, same age, with the same good diets and habits, same weight, and same position on the continuum, go into the hospital for surgery. One of them, however, at the nagging of a relative, brings along some vitamin and mineral supplements and takes them with every meal. The same surgeon performs the same surgical procedure on both people on the same day. Both operations proceed smoothly.

Ten days later the person who didn't take supplements goes home well. The person who took supplements, however, has already been home for three days.

Was the person who didn't take supplements getting "enough" vitamins and minerals? What did *more* vitamins and minerals do for the person who took supplements?

A final example: In 1948, Dr. Harold Chope started surveying the diets of 577 residents of San Mateo County, California. He kept records of what they ate, the amounts of certain vitamins in their diets, and their health. After six years, he analyzed his data to see if nutrition had anything to do with health and longevity.

Dr. Chope found that people with a higher-than-average intake of vitamins A, C, and niacin *did* tend to live longer than those with lower intakes. During the six years, there were over four times as many deaths among people getting *less* than 50 mg. of vitamin C as there were among people getting *more* than 50 mg. Vitamins had an effect on what kinds of diseases people suffered, too. People with high intakes of vitamin A had less disease of the nervous system, circulatory system, and respiratory system. People with high intakes of vitamin C had less disease of the circulatory system and digestive tract.[1]

Our position on the continuum is determined by an intricate system of supply and demand. If we merely want to stand still, maintain a certain status quo, and keep from slipping back into illness, we must meet certain nutritional demands. The eighteenth-century sailors who got scurvy on long sea voyages did so because their base requirement for vitamin C was not being supplied. Neither of the surgical patients in the second example above had scurvy. Their base requirements were met. But one of them supplied a demand for *optimum healing* that the other did not. The person who increases his or her vitamin-mineral supply, and experiences improved health or performance, is supplying a demand for optimum health.

What are vitamins and minerals? What roles do they play? How do they determine our position on the illness-health continuum?

In order for life to go on—in order for us to be able to walk, talk, think, play, work, eat, or do *anything* we do—every cell in the body must perform its own special function. Blood cells must carry nutrients, oxygen, and waste products; nerve cells must carry impulses; muscle cells must contract; etc.

The basic raw materials for these functions are the *macro-nutrients*: oxygen, water, protein, carbohydrates, and fats. Oxygen is, of course, the most basic requirement of the cells. The cells burn fuel for energy by combining it with oxygen, the way any furnace or engine does. If the cell's supply of oxygen is cut off, the cells die. If the supply is impaired, cell function is impaired too.

Oxygen is carried to the cells by means of *hemoglobin,* a protein in the red blood cells.

Water is also a necessary nutrient. Not only does water take part in many biochemical reactions and transport chemicals from one place to another within the body, but it is also *the* major component of the body.

Proteins are the "building blocks" of the body. All growth, repair, and maintenance requires proteins and cells, which are constructed from proteins. Proteins are large, complex molecules that contain nitrogen. There are over a thousand different proteins in the body. These are made up of different combinations of twenty smaller molecules called *amino acids.*

Of the twenty amino acids, the body can synthesize twelve, but cannot synthesize the remaining eight. These must be supplied in the diet. If all the eight essential amino acids are not present in the digestive tract at once, protein will not be synthesized, but will be broken down and used for energy, stored as fat, or excreted. Excess protein not required for tissue repair, growth, or maintenance is also either burned for energy or stored as fat.

Nutritional scientists estimate our protein requirements to be about eight tenths of a gram of protein per kilogram of body weight, which translates to about a third of a gram of protein for every pound of body weight. Illness, injury, trauma, severe stress, or extraordinary energy expenditure can boost the requirement for protein.

Carbohydrates are the starches and sugars that provide the body's main fuel, *glucose*. Except for lactose, a milk sugar, and ribose, a sugar found in animals' nucleic acid, all carbohydrates are produced by photosynthesis in plants. Carbohydrates are broken down in digestion into the simple sugars glucose, fructose, and galactose, which are all converted to glucose in the liver.

Glucose enters the bloodstream and is distributed to the body tissues where it serves as fuel. Excess glucose is stored in the liver and muscle tissues as *glycogen*, and mobilized for future needs. When tissue reserves of glycogen are filled to capacity, remaining excess glucose is converted to and stored as fat.

If no stored glycogen and fat are available when the body needs energy, the body will start to break down tissue proteins for fuel, much the same way the crew of an out-of-fuel steamboat will begin tearing apart and burning furniture, cargo, and expendable parts of the ship's structure in order to supply energy.

Fat was once thought of as merely the body's reserve energy supply. Fat *is* the most efficient way to store fuel for the body. But fats, or fatty acids, are also required for other metabolic and structural functions. Fats are necessary for the absorption and transport of fat-soluble vitamins, for example. Many hormones and other body fluids require fat for their synthesis. And *essential fatty acids*—of which there are three: linoleic acid, linolenic acid, and arachidonic acid—have been found to have some roles similar to those of the vitamins, as cofactors in many important biological reactions. Essential fatty acids have also been found to be an actual part of the structure of the cells. The body cannot synthesize essential fatty acids, so it needs a steady supply of them in the diet.

But the macronutrients aren't all that's needed. In order to do its job, every cell or system of cells also depends on certain chemicals or enzymes being in the right places at the right times, and in the right amounts, in order to carry out the many functions necessary to digesting and metabolizing the macronutrients. Many chain reactions must occur in the proper sequence. And all of these chain reactions depend on a supply of certain chemicals from outside the body called *micronutrients*, because they're supplied in minute quantities.

Think of it as a baseball game. The players are these necessary enzymes and chemicals. You must have enough players on the field before the game can go on. Every player depends on the other players, too. The pitcher pitches the ball, but if the catcher isn't there to catch it, you won't have much of a game. If the batter isn't there to try to hit the ball, the game is a waste of time, too. If the first baseman isn't there and the batter hits the ball to the shortstop, his team is in real trouble. Other players may be able to cover for missing or underperforming players, but they do so at the expense of their own performance. If the outfielders don't show up, you'll have some very tired infielders. And if the pitcher disappears in the middle of the game's most crucial inning, you've got no game at all!

Inside our bodies there are thousands of different baseball games being played for millions and millions of fans—the cells. These games are the metabolic processes involving proteins, carbohydrates, fats, water, and oxygen. If the games are in any way impaired—if some of the players are having off days, or simply don't show—the fans really suffer.

Some of these players—chemicals—are common everyday players. They live at the ballpark (that is, they are synthesized by the body) and always show up for the game. Others—the star players—have to be brought in from outside the park.

These star players are the vitamins and essential minerals. Without them, the game cannot be played, and the fans are the worse for it.

Vitamins are organic compounds that act as cofactors or regulators in metabolic processes crucial to life and cannot be synthesized by the body but must be supplied from outside. Before the term *vitamin* was coined, these chemicals were called *accessory factors*. In 1911 a researcher named Funk started calling them *vitamines* after his observation that the anti-beriberi factor he isolated from rice polishings was an *amine* (a chemical compound containing nitrogen).

Funk wanted to emphasize that these substances were more than accessories, that they were quite crucial to life, or *vital*. In 1920 the term *vitamin* was created as a compromise, since not all the substances were amines.

As new factors or vitamins were discovered, letters of the alphabet were used to distinguish them. And as nutritional scientists discovered more and more life processes that depended upon vitamins, the list grew longer and longer. Actually, many substances thought to be new vitamins were later found to be old vitamins discovered in an additional function.

For example, it was thought that a single substance was responsible for the many functions attributed to what is now called the *B complex* of vitamins. As more and more distinct chemicals were isolated and identified, they were given subscripts B_1, B_2, B_3, etc. This became confusing because there was no order to the naming of new B vitamins. Many of the "new" B vitamins turned out to be old ones discovered in a new function.

Furthermore, the B vitamins are not really part of a *complex* at all. Although they are found together in many foods, and many of their functions do interrelate or overlap, they are chemically unrelated. The B vitamins are generally involved in cellular oxidation, the process by which the cell burns fuel to provide energy, and in the digestion and absorption of food and nutrients.

Overlapping of functions is not uncommon among vitamins. The critical functions of the cells require many steps, and vitamins and minerals are involved all along the way. If one particular step is blocked by a deficiency in one nutrient, the effect on the cell or system of cells may be the same as if some other step in the same process were blocked. If the first baseman isn't there to catch the shortstop's throw, the effect is much the same as if the shortstop weren't there to throw it.

The vitamins aren't the only factors or star players that must be brought in from outside the park. Essential minerals must be, too. Minerals differ from vitamins in that they are *not* compounds but *elements*, which cannot be broken down any further or constructed from other chemicals, as can vitamins. Minerals perform some of the same types of functions as vitamins—as essential cofactors in biochemical reactions. But they also serve as structural components in tissues—such as calcium and phosphorus in bone—and as raw materials or central participants in biochemical reactions. Sodium, for example, is required to pump water in and out of cells. And iron is the part of the hemoglobin that carries oxygen to the cells.

Minerals that are needed in minute amounts are called *trace minerals*. Those like calcium and phosphorus, which are required in large amounts for use as raw materials, are called *bulk minerals*.

When the vitamins or minerals don't show up for the game, the enzyme systems and other chemical reactions that depend on them falter and grind to a halt. The body cannot synthesize its own supply, so it loses the ability to utilize food, burn fuel, and carry out biochemical functions.

If enough players are absent, life ends. If they are undersupplied—if they show up but are having a bad day— life may go on, but in a weaker, suboptimal, semidiseased way.

We need them all there in full force, playing their best game, before we can hope to play ours.

Each vitamin and mineral plays a different position. Most

play more than one; many play dozens. (The life game has hundreds of positions.) In each chapter we'll consider what each vitamin or mineral does and point out the biochemical games that depend on it.

We'll look at what happens when demand exceeds supply, which biochemical functions and body systems suffer the most. And we'll learn the symptoms of a deficiency. Even though these symptoms will often be extreme, you'll want to know them because a person can suffer lesser versions of extreme symptoms when a deficiency is only marginal—when the demand only slightly outstrips the supply.

You can't expect too much purity of effect when it comes to nutrient deficiencies. Nor can you expect absolute uniformity from species to species, or from individual to individual. Differences at the cellular level can be great enough to lend substantial variety to deficiency symptoms. One person's riboflavin need may be greater in the skin and mucous membranes. Another's may be in the adrenal glands. Still another's might be in the heart muscle.

Doctors and nutritionists are finding many new uses and potential uses for vitamins and minerals. They find, for instance, that low levels of certain nutrients are associated with certain diseases. This is the first step in a series of investigations that eventually leads to experiments attempting to find out if the nutrients involved can help prevent or treat the diseases.

Sometimes, the investigative path has not yet reached the point where people are being helped. The experiments may involve animals, or biochemical measurements without actual human therapeutic trials. This information is still very useful because it gives strong indications of ways in which vitamins and minerals might keep people moving toward optimum health.

One of the questions uppermost in people's minds is *How much of each vitamin and mineral do we need?* This is a question no one can completely answer for anyone else, because it depends on how close to optimum health a person wants to get and how much of each nutrient it takes to help that particular person get there.

Everyone eats different amounts and kinds of food; everyone has different levels and types of stress; everyone has different biochemical ball games going on inside, with the players all playing at different speeds and effectiveness.

Although the question *How much should I take?* cannot be answered with any certainty for all people, there is a lot of information that can help people decide for themselves. Let's start by giving the RDAs (recommended daily allowances) for each nutrient.

The RDAs are determined by a committee of scientists and nutritionists of the National Academy of Sciences. Like any other committee, they meet with "witnesses" who testify as to how high or low the requirements should be set, and for which substances they should be determined. And, like all committees, they are subject to the same influences of fellowship, corruption, and sincere dedication.

It's a genuine temptation to convene the committee and charge them with determining the RDA for oxygen. Once they've done that, each member should be fitted with an airtight breather which would be supplied with exactly the RDA for oxygen. No more, no less. Then, all the people who believe the RDAs are adequate should also be fitted with the breathers. The rest of us could enjoy that wasteful bounty of air all around us. Anyone who believes a committee could determine, with any accuracy, the needs of an incredibly diverse range of people, conditions, needs, stresses, biochemical factors, etc. should put their lungs where their mouth is and not flinch at this degree of trust.

RDAs have a function, and that function is to give the food industry a reference point in determining how much of the various nutrients are contained in their products. A manufacturer of bread, for example, wants to be able to tell you what percentage of the RDA for certain nutrients is contained in his bread. You can immediately see the possibility for abuse, since it's in the food industry's best interests to keep the RDAs as low as possible and keep the list of required nutrients as small as possible. No food processor wants to have to print on the label that ninety percent of the nutrients have been removed from his product! He wants to be able to say it contains fifty percent of the RDA for this one and that one and forget the rest. He wants to be able to "fortify" the product with some cheap vitamins and say it contains a hundred percent of a few—and ignore the twenty-two others that were removed in processing.

But our body doesn't forget the rest. Nature isn't bound by the committee's decisions.

Some people can get along with the RDAs of the vitamins and minerals. Some can probably get along with less. Many undoubtedly need more. The variations in requirements reported by scientists are too great to presume that any committee could determine the needs of a diverse population, and thus the RDAs bear little or no relation to nutritional reality.

For each nutrient, there are factors which determine our individual needs, and we'll have a closer look at those. Basically, three things must happen before a vitamin or mineral can do the body any good. First, it must be absorbed from the stomach or intestine. Second, it must be transported to the site(s) where it is used—the cells. Third, it must be made usable to the cells by undergoing specific chemical transformations or bondings with other chemicals. It's important to know these three necessities, because at any one of these points a multitude of factors can determine how well a nutrient does its job. There may be varying levels of absorption in the gut; there may be defects or abnormal demands that route nutrients to different places in the body—or out of the body. There may be metabolic irregularities that hamper the cells' use of the nutrients even though they're available.

These factors result in a wide range of individual requirements. In some cases, where metabolic defects are severe, super or *mega* doses of vitamins or minerals are required to force a slow game into motion, or force enough of a nutrient into the bloodstream to do some good. Also, a person may need more vitamins or minerals simply to meet the demand set by his or her personal combination of stress and biochemical individuality.

Does that mean we all have to take vitamin and mineral supplements in order to be healthy? This is another question no one can answer for you.

A lot of people don't like the idea of taking nutritional supplements because they feel they can get all the vitamins and minerals they need from their food. Theoretically, this should be possible. But it's not as simple or as easy as many people think it is. Furthermore, there are many factors that interfere. The most important factor, of course, is a person's individual needs. Considering the wide range of individual requirements, there will be people who get along just fine with no supplements and an average diet, just as there will be people who need more than any diet can possibly supply. In the middle are people with moderate or "normal" needs, which means they need more than an average (poor) diet provides, but not so much that a diet of the *right* foods can't fulfill their needs. If you are the theoretical person who can get by without watching your diet at all, good for you.

People in the second category are people who have clinically obvious deficiencies, people who are ill (either chronically or acutely), people who have malabsorption syndromes, and people who merely have greater biochemical requirements.

But those of us in the middle aren't nearly as sure of our specific needs.

Maybe you're taking vitamins and minerals now and don't notice any difference. Or maybe you're not taking supplements and wonder if you should, despite the fact that you feel OK.

Let's start with the assumption that there exists a diet that will provide all your nutritional requirements. First of all, it would have to be mostly, if not all, natural foods. Processed foods are totally unreliable as sources of most of the required vitamins and minerals. Too much is removed during processing and not enough is put back, and substances are added that further lower the quality of the food.

Once you eliminate processed and junk food from your diet and start using natural foods, you're still not home free. You never know, for sure, where your natural foods came from and under what conditions they were produced. These are important factors because they determine the levels of nutrients. Many of the trace minerals are undersupplied in large areas of farmland. Modern agricultural practices have a way of replenishing the soil with only the nutrients that produce a big crop. A big crop isn't necessarily a nutritious crop. Even if you grow all your own food, the variations in nutritional value can be enormous, owing to differences in sunlight, storage time, preservation methods, time of harvest.

If you *cook* most of your food, you should immediately stop thinking you can get by without a supplement, because cooking destroys significant quantities of many nutrients. So even if you grow your own food, and you're sure there are plenty of minerals in your soil, you still have to be careful what you do with the food between the times it comes from the earth and goes into your body.

If you rely on others to prepare your food, chances are good your requirements aren't being met. Institutional food lives up to its reputation as mediocre. Malnutrition is common in hospitals, usually despite the best efforts of dedicated dieticians. School lunches must cater to other considerations besides nutritional quality, and surveys have found them frequently inadequate. And although you may pay twenty dollars for a restaurant meal, do you know where the food came from and how it was stored and prepared?

It's just too much trouble to check out all your food that way. Here are some general guidelines to follow: Eat lots of fresh fruits and vegetables, mostly raw; lean meats and fish; whole grains and cereals; small amounts of dairy products; as little fat as possible.

It's hard to stick to these rules, especially if you don't grow any of your own food.

There are more factors. Prescription drugs raise requirements. Many people *can't* avoid them, but you should try to. There's no common prescription drug that doesn't interfere with at least one nutrient.

Pollutants raise requirements. Lead, cadmium, ozone . . . even if you grow all your own food and fulfill requirements that might have been enough when our body evolved, the fact is the human body evolved in clean air and water. Many of the body's defensive reactions to the poisons in the environment raise nutritional requirements, as described in later chapters.

Stress raises requirements, too. The caveman had to cope with sabertoothed tigers and a host of natural threats. But the cave dwellers didn't live in a world that kept their fight-or-flight mechanism on alert most of their waking hours. Taking vitamin supplements will not fully protect anyone against the ravages of modern life. But there are unavoidable stresses, plus the stresses we don't choose to avoid because they are either pleasurable, stimulating, or necessary. And it's nice to know we can help the body prepare for and deal with these when the time comes.

One last consideration is that the level of nutrition necessary for survival will not necessarily be adequate for optimum health. In the natural world, organisms generally cope with imperfect nutrition. The caveman probably did, too. There are a lot of things we don't *have* to do which, undone, will not seriously threaten our usefulness to the survival of the race. Most of the serious effects of marginal nutritional deficiencies don't show up until we're past the age where most people have children. But optimum health at any age may be a luxury that requires optimum nutrition, among other things.

Once we have an idea of how much we need, we want to know *Where do we get it?* We'll list the best natural food sources of each vitamin and mineral and briefly describe what kinds of supplements are available.

People have other questions about vitamins and minerals. For example, some vitamins are water soluble and some are fat soluble. The fat soluble vitamins (A, D, E, K) dissolve in fat and in substances that dissolve fat. They're usually found in the fatty portions of foods. They are absorbed along with fats in the gastrointestinal tract and are stored in the fatty parts of the liver and other tissues.

Water-soluble vitamins dissolve in water. They are not stored to any great extent in the body since water flushes through the system quite rapidly. Any condition that steps up the flow of water through the body—stress, exertion, sweating, diuretic drugs, diarrhea—can result in abnormal loss of these vitamins.

There are other common questions about vitamins and minerals. People want to know how they can determine how much supplementation they need. They want to know when to take their supplements. They want to know if natural vitamins are superior to synthetic. They want to know how to buy supplements.

The answers to these questions require giving more information than an introduction can handle. You should first know more about the individual vitamins and minerals and how they affect health before attempting to figure out which supplements you should take, if any. For this reason, the final chapter of the book has been reserved for these questions, "The Eight Most Asked Questions about Vitamins and Minerals." At least, these are the eight most common *after* the questions answered in this chapter.

There is one more thing to add to this introduction: Vitamins and minerals can't solve all the health problems in life, nor are they the only factors that can move us closer to optimum health. Faddism, or vitamin hysteria, comes from expecting vitamins and minerals to be the answer to everything that can go wrong with health. This attitude is every bit as foolish as denying that vitamins and minerals can do anything at all to help us improve our health. As a matter of fact, that denial is also a form of vitamin hysteria.

There's nothing faddish about expecting vitamins and minerals to be effective tools for improving health, performance, and well-being. Some of the studies cited in this book are more than a half-century old. Doctors were using many of these nutritional therapies long before most of the current drugs or surgical procedures were developed.

Everybody knows somebody who has been helped by some dietary change, whether it's eating less meat and more fruits and vegetables or taking a handful of supplements every day. If you want to move closer to the optimum health end of the illness-health continuum, nutrition should definitely be one area of your life you should examine. This book will help you do that.

section 1
VITAMINS

1

Vitamin A

You're strolling the last couple of blocks home on one of those winter evenings when it gets dark early. Suddenly the street lights flicker and die, and you're staring down two blackened blocks between you and the safety of your own home.

Or the lighted freeway suddenly runs out of construction funds and spits you onto a country road that might as well be the middle of the Black Forest for all the moonlight that filters through the trees. To make matters worse, every oncoming car's headlights flare up at you, pass, and plunge you into even deeper darkness.

Or maybe you're sitting in your favorite easy chair with a mystery novel. It's too scary to put down and go to bed. But then the main fuse blows, and you've got to go down into the cellar to replace it. However, the batteries in your flashlight are dead.

For many people these situations are too terrifying to even

think about. Others would press on almost as if nothing had happened although the sudden darkness would certainly be momentarily disorienting. The difference is that for some people, the darkened street would become visible again before they had gone ten steps, the darkness of the country road would spread like a curtain parted by the car's headlights, and the light of a candle would be more than enough to guide the way to the fusebox.

Some people's eyes adjust to low-light situations faster than others. That's a fact. But what's also a fact is that vitamin A can determine how fast your eyes adjust to darkness. *Visual purple*, the pigment in the retina required for adaptation to darkness, depends on a constant supply of vitamin A for regeneration. So sensitive is this requirement that night blindness is the first easily recognizable symptom that your vitamin A supply is not fulfilling the demand. So you might think you're as close to optimal health as you can be. But if your eyes don't adjust well to the darkness, you might be able to get even closer.

WHAT VITAMIN A DOES

Vitamin A is important for a lot more than whether our eyes adjust to the darkness. It plays a crucial role in protecting at least three of our senses; it is absolutely necessary if we're to fight off infections; and it promises to be of great benefit in battling skin problems, abnormally heavy menstrual bleeding, and cancer.

Vitamin A's chemical name, *retinol*, is derived from its function in eyesight. A healthy *retina* must contain a minimum amount of vitamin A because the vitamin actively participates in the chemical process by which light stimulates the rods and cones into sending sight messages to the brain.

More than the eyes depend on vitamin A. *Epithelial tissues*, the layers of tissue covering an organ or an entire organism (such as the skin or mucous membranes), depend on vitamin A for healthy structure and function. Vitamin A is also required for the proper growth and maintenance of the bones and teeth. Some current research is attempting to find out more about vitamin A's suspected role in the structure and function of all biologic membranes, the "border" membranes between cells.

There is some evidence from animal studies that vitamin A may act as an *antioxidant,* which means it prevents tissues from combining with oxygen too rapidly. Every cell needs a certain amount of oxygen to survive, of course. But when the material of the cell itself combines with oxygen, the structure and function of the cell suffers. Oxidation of cellular and intracellular tissues appears to be a common factor in aging and in many diseases.

Vitamin A is also necessary for the proper structure and function of the adrenal glands, which control our response to stress.[1] When the body is under stress, the adrenal glands secrete hormones which orchestrate the various organs necessary to deal with this stress. Keep in mind that our stress response evolved when stress invariably meant physical danger. So even if few contemporary stresses can de dealt with by force, the body still prepares for a *fight* or a *flight.* The heart rate speeds up, the blood pressure rises, and the conversion of fat and proteins to energy increases in order to make more energy available for the muscles.

WHAT HAPPENS WHEN VITAMIN A DEMAND EXCEEDS SUPPLY

The first sign that the body needs more vitamin A than it's getting is the loss of night vision. There may be biochemical signs long before night vision begins to suffer, however. A recent study revealed that *anemia* often occurs first—even before blood levels of the vitamin drop to so-called deficient levels. The subjects of this experiment were middle-aged men, not people you'd expect to suffer from anemia. Furthermore, they were given a diet containing almost *twice* the Recommended Daily Allowance for iron. Still, their blood levels of iron *dropped,* and the ability of their blood to deliver oxygen to the cells was severely diminished. Massive doses of iron were able to alleviate the situation somewhat, but only for a limited time. As soon as vitamin A was restored to their diet, however, their anemia went away.[2]

Since all the cells of the body need oxygen to survive and function correctly, it's not difficult to understand how devastating a deficiency of vitamin A can be. That stress response we call upon so many times each day makes heavy demands on the adrenal glands and the oxygen-carrying ability of the blood. If the vitamin A needed for these functions is supplied in marginal amounts, optimal health is impossible. And since most doctors are not trained to recognize any anemia except iron-deficiency anemia, it's interesting to speculate how many people who are troubled with fatigue from a suboptimal intake of vitamin A are mistakenly given iron supplements to do the job.

If you know of (or *are*) such a person, the best course of action is to examine yourself for the visible symptoms of vitamin A deficiency. Besides loss of adaptation to darkness, the classic symptom of vitamin A deficiency is a *drying out,* or *hyperkeratinization,* of the skin and mucous membranes. In its early stages, hyperkeratinization resembles "goose bumps that won't go away," and proceeds until the skin takes on a horny, rough texture. This drying out and toughening of the tissues can be a serious problem when it extends to membranes that are normally moist and soft, such as the mucous membranes that line the mouth, respiratory tract, genitourinary tract, gastrointestinal tract, eyes, and certain glands (the endocrine, salivary, sebaceous, and lacrimal glands). Loss of the senses of taste and smell are two early signs of hyperkeratinization of the mucous membranes.[3]

When this drying out occurs in the eyes, night blindness is the first, relatively minor, symptom. If the deficiency gets worse, *xerosis,* or drying, of the cornea and conjunctiva occurs. Both of these effects are more serious than night blindness, but they are also reversible if adequate vitamin A is supplied. If the vitamin A deficiency continued to worsen, however, *xerophthalmia*—irreversible corneal damage and scarring—results. The cornea starts to deteriorate, intraocular pressure can be lost, and the lens can be expelled, losing vision for good. Worldwide, xerophthalmia is one of the major causes of blindness, affecting as many as 200,000 children every year.[4]

CAN MORE VITAMIN A IN MY DIET DO ANY GOOD?

If you have trouble adapting to the dark, more vitamin A in your diet may help. A Florida doctor randomly tested 100 people and found 26 whose night vision was deficient. He then gave all who were night-blind a daily supplement of 25,000 units of vitamin A. Within a week and a half, ninety percent of the people "responded favorably."[5]

You may feel that you never really need your night vision. So why worry about getting enough vitamin A to maintain it? Remember, however, that night blindness is only the first sign that your vitamin A supply is not meeting the demand. Chances are good that you're moving in the wrong direction on the illness-health continuum if your vitamin A supply isn't adequate to maintain your night vision.

Vitamin A and Infection

For example, nothing cramps your style like an infection. Try to do your best work when your head aches, your nose runs, and your insides ache from coughing. If your vitamin A supply is suboptimal, you're leaving yourself open to unnecessary infections, because vitamin A is crucial to the body's defenses. The most frequent cause of death in animals deprived of vitamin A is infection.[6] You don't have to be *deprived* to suffer the consequences, however. The mucous membranes—which are dependent upon vitamin A for their structure and function—are the body's first line of defense against infections. When these membranes dry out, they allow invading organisms to take hold and multiply. *Mucocutane-ous candidiasis,* a fungus that attacks the skin, mouth, and vagina, is one such organism. Doctors have found that vitamin A levels are lower than normal in people suffering this infection.[7]

Vitamin A's role in protecting us against infection extends much deeper. Doctors have tested this by injecting mice with dangerous bacteria responsible for pneumonia, meningitis, and a wide range of other infections. Without fail, the mice receiving extra vitamin A fare better than the animals who get low or normally "adequate" amounts. In one experiment, the blood of the vitamin A–treated animals was still sterile after all the other animals had been killed by the infection.[8]

The fact that vitamin A seems to exert a protective effect against a wide range of bacteria and viruses suggests that it is actually boosting the body's own defenses. High blood levels of the vitamin don't simply kill the invading organisms, because when researchers place vitamin A in test tube cultures of bacteria, there is no destructive effect. Some researchers believe that vitamin A stimulates the *macrophages,* which are large cells the body mobilizes to devour invading organisms.

When a specific nutrient is mobilized from its storage sites in the body during a particular stress, it's reasonable to assume that the nutrient has an important role in the body's response to the stress. This response will sometimes result in higher-than-normal blood or tissue levels of the nutrient. When *lower*-than-normal levels of a nutrient are measured, however, the nutrient may also be required to keep the body moving toward optimum health. Larger-than-normal amounts of the nutrient may be required to keep blood and tissue levels where they ought to be, and the body's stores may have already been used up.

Measurements of blood levels or bodily utilization of a nutrient are often the only way researchers can examine the nutrient's role in human disease processes. You can't expect too many experiments where people are injected with dangerous microorganisms and varying levels of vitamin A. But you can expect to find studies where people suffering from various diseases are measured for nutrient levels. In one case, researchers demonstrated that children with rheumatic fever had low blood levels of vitamin A. And when their fever intensified, their vitamin A levels dropped still further. The same researchers went a step further—but with *animals*. They injected rats with inflammatory substances and measured their blood and liver levels of vitamin A. In all cases, the vitamin A levels decreased sharply when the inflammation took hold.[9]

Vitamin A and Healing

In order for a wound to heal, new collagen must be formed and linked to hold new tissue together. That linking is dependent upon vitamin A. In animal studies, vitamin A supplements enabled wounded rats to heal faster and become stronger than rats not given extra vitamin A. The rats given extra vitamin A also gained twice as much weight, an indication that the vitamin A was helping the healing process and boosting the body's overall response to a severe stress.[10]

Vitamin A has a beneficial effect upon human healing as well. Antiinflammatory drugs, such as cortisone, are among the most commonly prescribed drugs. But one of the unfortunate side effects of these drugs is the suppression of the healing process. Vitamin A, taken orally or applied *topically* (directly to the wound), can restore normal healing. In one case a five-year-old girl taking cortisone had a sore on her foot that absolutely refused to heal. After six weeks she was given vitamin A ointment, which was applied to the wound. The sore healed within ten days.[11]

Vitamin A and Heavy Menstrual Bleeding

Vitamin A's beneficial effect on healing applied to other circumstances besides actual wounds. Heavy menstrual bleeding not only drives women to distraction, but also to unnecessary hysterectomies. There are other causes for *menorrhagia,* but once those other causes are ruled out, there's a good chance vitamin A could be the answer. Doctors have found that women who suffer abnormally heavy or extended menstrual flow from no other apparent cause seem to have low blood levels of vitamin A. Many women who suffer this dysfunction from other causes also have low vitamin A levels. In one study, when 52 menorrhagic women were given 30,000 units of vitamin A twice a day for 35 days, 23 were restored to normal, 14 reported improvement in their condition, and 12 did not return for follow-up examination—usually an indication that the medication helped.[12]

Vitamin A and Cancer

There is more than enough evidence to establish that vitamin A plays an important role in fighting cancer. Epidemiological studies, in which large numbers of people with various forms of cancer were tested, have demonstrated that vitamin A deficiencies are associated with cancer of the stomach, nasopharynx, and respiratory tract.[13] A Norwegian study involving over 8000 men found that high incidence of lung cancer was associated with low intake of vitamin A. This relationship held true at all levels of cigarette smoking. Men whose vitamin A intake was moderate or high were found to have a low likelihood of cancer.[14]

Many precancerous conditions are similar, if not identical, to some of the effects of a vitamin A deficiency. The mucous membranes which dry out in a deficiency happen to be common sites for many cancers. Hyperkeratinization, the "drying out" that occurs in a vitamin A deficiency, is a common feature in *squamous metaplasia*—an abnormal, precancerous scaliness of the tissue. Vitamin A levels in the blood plasma of people with squamous cell carcinoma of the mouth and oropharynx were measured and compared to levels in people without the disease. More than half of the cancer patients had deficient or low levels of vitamin A, compared to from three to seventeen percent of the controls. The researchers who carried out this experiment point out that not only are the lesions of vitamin A deficiency potentially precancerous, but that these lesions resemble those induced by cancer-causing chemicals.[15]

Apparently vitamin A fights cancer the same way it helps the body fight infections—by boosting the power of the immune defense system. We know that in a vitamin A deficiency, the immune system is compromised. And we know that low vitamin A levels correspond not only to the incidence of cancer but also to the progression of tumors. Many researchers believe that our bodies must *constantly* deal with low levels of cancerous activity which is not only spontaneously generated within the body but also stimulated by cancer-causing agents in the environment. If this cancerous activity increases beyond the immune system's ability to handle it or if the immune system is weakened by any of a number of factors, cancer occurs.[16]

Tests with animals have demonstrated that cancer-causing chemicals are more effective in the presence of a vitamin A deficiency. Conversely, vitamin A has been found to prevent, retard, or reverse the growth of skin cancers on mice. Certain anticancer drugs are more effective if vitamin A is included in the therapy.[17]

In a National Cancer Institute study, vitamin A substantially reduced the effects on mice of a potent chemical cause of breast cancer. At "normal" doses of the chemical, none of the vitamin A-protected mice got breast cancer, while twenty-seven percent of the unprotected mice did. At much higher doses of the carcinogen, twenty-seven percent and fifty-three percent of the vitamin A-protected mice got cancer, compared to forty-eight and eighty-seven percent of the others.[18]

There is one report of the effect of vitamin A treatment on human cancer. Massive doses amounting to at least 30 million units were given to nine men with inoperable lung cancer. Two of the men died because their disease was already too widespread. A third man died after showing signs of a complete remission, which led doctors to speculate that he died from either the toxicity of the vitamin A or from the products of tumor disintegration. But the effect of vitamin A treatment on the rest of the men was remarkable. Tumor progression was either slowed or stopped. There was no further spread of cancer to other parts of the body. And the men's psychological condition also improved during the treatment program. The researchers noted that the men's immune system had apparently been stimulated, because their lymphocyte (white blood cell) activity increased. And giving vitamin A to other cancer patients who, unlike the nine men, were also receiving anticancer drugs and radiation therapy, also boosted their immune systems. This is an important effect, since the conventional means of fighting cancer usually depress the immune system. It's also important because it means that extra vitamin A in the diet can help *prevent* cancer from taking hold in the first place.

Vitamin A and Retinitis Pigmentosa

Retinitis pigmentosa is a frequently hereditary condition in which the retina becomes abnormally pigmented and atrophied. The field of vision gradually shrinks. This disease has not traditionally been associated with vitamin A deficiency. Yet some enterprising researchers did find that people with the disease happened to have low blood levels of the vitamin. Another group of doctors tried supplements of vitamin A on people with retinitis pigmentosa after checking their blood levels of vitamin A and finding them "strikingly low." The patients were given 50,000 units of vitamin A each day. Their blood levels rose rapidly and their gradual shrinkage of vision was either slowed up, stopped, or reversed. Vitamin A had the greatest effect on people under thirty. There were no toxic symptoms at that level of supplementation.[19]

Vitamin A and Prenatal Development

A vitamin A deficiency during pregnancy can have disastrous effects upon the developing fetus. Understandably, most of the experimental work done to reveal these effects is performed with animals rather than people. For example, sows give birth to eyeless piglets when their diet is deficient in vitamin A. Cleft palate and lip, extra ears, and kidney defects are also noted. When the same sows are fed adequate vitamin A during subsequent pregnancies, all members of their litters are normal.

Requirements for most nutrients rise during pregnancy. Rats will appear healthy, with no signs of deficiency, at a certain level of intake. But to produce healthy offspring, they need about 20 times as much vitamin A. Otherwise, litters are born with malformed hearts, blood vessels, and teeth.[20]

Just because *rats* need 20 times their normal vitamin A intake in order to have healthy offspring doesn't necessarily mean humans need 20 times their normally adequate amount. But it does suggest that pregnant women do need more than what will normally keep them moving toward optimum health.

HOW MUCH VITAMIN A DO WE NEED?

The RDA (recommended daily dietary allowance) for vitamin A is 5000 IU (international units) for men, 4000 IU for women, 1400 for infants, 2000–3300 for children, 5000 for pregnant women, and 6000 for lactating mothers. Individual requirements for vitamins and minerals vary greatly. In one experiment in which the vitamin A requirement for rats was to be determined, the range was so varied that the researchers could not arrive at a definite figure. There were healthy, vigorous animals in *all* groups, including the group that got *no vitamin A at all* for the length of the study![21]

It's quite reasonable to assume that human requirements for vitamin A vary greatly, too. There are too many factors that can get in the way of a person's getting an adequate supply. For example, heat is not destructive of vitamin A, but oxidation is. And heat increases the rate of oxidation. So cooking at high temperatures for a long time, with subsequent exposure to the air during storage, can substantially reduce vitamin A content of foods. Furthermore, vitamin A in plants is not as available to human digestion unless a small amount of cooking has softened the cell walls that make up the vegetable. Smashing, blending, or liquifying vegetables can help make more vitamin A available by breaking down many of the cell walls. Vitamin A content of vegetables will vary greatly, too, according to the condition of the soil, the amount of sunlight, and other factors.

Everyone does not necessarily need to take vitamin A supplements. But you cannot assume your diet is providing enough of the vitamin to keep you moving toward the optimum health end of the continuum. If you eat in fast-food restaurants much of the time, for example, you should be aware of the study which found that typical fast-food meals failed to supply an adequate supply of vitamin A to meet the RDA.[22]

Many chemicals we come in contact with every day are a drain on our body's store of vitamin A. We've already seen how steroid drugs raise the body's requirement, since it takes supplementation to restore normal healing powers. Not everyone takes steroid drugs, naturally. But there are few of us who don't take some amount of *polychlorinated biphenyl* (PCB) into our body every day. This toxic industrial chemical has been in use—and abuse—for almost fifty years. Because of the way pollutants manage to spread out through the food chain, chances are we're all getting *some* of this chemical, which inhibits growth and enlarges the liver.

Vitamin A detoxifies PCB. Rats fed a vitamin A-deficient diet with added PCB were more hurt by the poison than rats fed "adequate" amounts of vitamin A. But rats fed "extra" vitamin A were hardly affected at all by PCB. Obviously, the word "adequate" takes on new meaning in some situations. What was an adequate amount to maintain health under unstressed conditions was not adequate as soon as some stress started pushing the organism away from optimum health. And since common poisons such as sodium benzoate, nitrites, aflatoxin, DDT, and dieldrin are also known to affect the metabolism of vitamin A, there are many more situations which, like PCB, raise the level that is "adequate."[23]

Is there any evidence of widespread deficiency of vitamin A? In developing countries, vitamin A deficiencies are widespread and severe enough to blind thousands of children every year. In developed countries, deficiencies that severe are quite rare. But that doesn't mean everyone is getting a supply adequate to maintain or move toward optimum health. The Ten-State Nutrition Survey found that ten percent of all Americans weren't getting the RDA of vitamin A. In addition to these 20 million people, there are presumably many millions more who may be getting the RDA set by the government but who aren't getting the required amount set by their own bodies' stresses.

Some specific groups of people often constitute "ghettoes" of malnutrition. One study, for example, found that forty percent of a sample of middle-class old people were not getting the RDA of vitamin A.[24]

These figures suggest that millions of people are not supplied enough vitamin A in their diet to maintain or improve their health—millions of people who are not supplying a basic nutritional demand. This further implies that many millions of people could move closer to optimum health simply by raising the vitamin A content in their diet.

CAN WE GET TOO MUCH VITAMIN A?

This is an important question because vitamin A is usually one of the first vitamins mentioned when vitamin toxicity is discussed. Because any amount of the vitamin that the body can't immediately use is stored rather than excreted, vitamin A can build up to potentially toxic levels. However, the margin of safety is quite large.

To produce toxic symptoms in rats, for instance, the animals must be given 1000 times more than the usual nutritional need. In human adults, several *million* units are required—and that dosage must continue for *months*—before the symptoms of toxicity show up. Infants can be poisoned, however, with a single dose of about 350,000 IU.[25]

This information should not be used as a justification to take hundreds of thousands of units of vitamin A every day. The range of requirements swings both ways. Some sensitive individuals may take prolonged doses of no more than ten times the RDA before toxicity results.[26] So there is no simple answer to the question of how much is safe.

In clinical reports where high doses are routinely used, only the very highest doses (used in the treatment of cancer) produced any signs of toxicity. And there are reports of Antarctic explorers succumbing to hypervitaminosis A after eating dog or polar bear livers, which are extremely high in vitamin A.[27] But even in these cases, it took many days for the symptoms to progress from mild to bad to worse. In one study, doctors administered 150,000 IU of vitamin A daily to a large number of heart patients and observed no toxic symptoms during the study, which went on for six months.[28]

Though the risks of toxicity are not nearly so great as many people imagine, you should be aware of the *symptoms* of toxicity. As with many vitamins and minerals, the symptoms of getting too much vitamin A often resemble the symptoms of not getting enough.

If you take in too much carotene (vitamin A precursor supplied by vegetables) over a period of time, your skin will take on a yellow tint. Prolonged excessive intake of vitamin A can result in loss of hair, nausea, headache, drying and peeling of the skin, general pruritis, fatigue, loss of appetite, muscle weakness, bone and joint pain, bone fragility, and enlargement of the liver and spleen. There is a small amount of evidence that vitamin E lessens the toxic effects of vitamin A, but the mechanism is not known and the protective effect is not reliably established.[29]

Some researchers did attempt to answer the question *How much is best?* by surveying over a thousand dentists and their wives about their health and vitamin A intake. They found that as the vitamin A levels in the diet rose, so did the health of the respondents. Those who reported a daily intake of 33,000 IU apparently had the fewest symptoms and health complaints.[30] This study attempted to answer a complicated question in a simple way. You should not assume that 33,000 IU is the best daily intake of vitamin A for you. You may need more, or less, to supply your own demands for optimal health.

SOURCES OF VITAMIN A

Vitamin A is a fat-soluble vitamin. That doesn't necessarily mean you must eat a lot of fatty foods to get vitamin A. Provitamin A, or carotene, exists in abundance in the yellow and orange pigments of many fruits and vegetables and is converted to vitamin A in the intestine. It does help, however, if a little fat is present in the gut when the vitamin is ingested. And if there are any conditions which interfere with fat absorption, absorption of the vitamin will also be inhibited. Such conditions include chronic diarrhea, biliary and pancreatic dysfunction, celiac disease, or the consumption of mineral oil. Once the vitamin is absorbed, it's stored in the liver and other fatty portions of the body.

Preformed vitamin A is available only from animal sources, the principal one being liver. Egg yolk and dairy products are also good sources. Vegetable sources of carotene include dark-green leafy vegetables, deep yellow vegetables, and tomatoes.

Vitamin A supplements are available in a wide range of dosages in both natural and synthetic forms. Water-soluble forms are available for people with digestive problems which interfere with fat absorption. Natural vitamin A from fish liver oils is usually priced competitively with synthetic forms.

2

Thiamine (B₁)

If your car runs out of gas, you've got a problem. But if it sputters and stalls and generally acts as if it's running out of gas when the tank is full, you've got an even bigger problem. Some internal defect is preventing the fuel from doing its job.

Likewise, if you go without eating for a day or so, you may find yourself too fatigued to carry on a normal day's business. You've got a problem, but one which you can easily solve by "refueling." On the other hand, what do you do if your tank is full—if you're eating plenty of food—and you still find yourself "running out of gas" in the middle of the day?

If you were a car, it would be easy just to tear down your engine until the offending parts were found, replace the parts, and speed away. But we're not cars, and although surgeons might argue otherwise, it's not practical to disassemble us every time we've got a problem.

We are like a car, however, in that when we feel and act as if we're "out of gas" even though the tank is full, the chances are something is preventing the fuel from doing its job. In our bodies, the fuel is *sugar*, not gasoline. But while the car needs gasoline which has been refined from oil, its natural state, our body prefers to do its fuel refining itself. The body takes carbohydrates and changes them into sugar, which is burned by the cells for energy. In a car, there are two chemicals—gas and air—which are manipulated by various mechanical parts. But in the body, the basic two chemicals—sugar and oxygen— are manipulated by dozens of biochemical "parts," the enzymes and coenzymes that carry out biochemical reactions.

WHAT THIAMINE DOES

Thiamine happens to be one of the coenzymes which plays a vital role in the energy-producing process. Its primary function is as part of a coenzyme system that makes possible carbohydrate metabolism. You can think of thiamine as one of the spark plugs that keeps the energy-producing functions of the body going. Since thiamine also plays a role in the excitation of nerves, it compares to the electrical part of a car's ignition system—which *sparks* the car to life.

WHAT HAPPENS WHEN
THIAMINE DEMAND EXCEEDS SUPPLY

When more fuel than the spark plugs can handle is injected into the firing chamber of an automobile engine, the engine misfires. Eventually, the plugs become fouled with waste products of the incomplete combustion. The same thing happens when thiamine is supplied in quantities which are inadequate for the energy demands of the body. The waste products which "foul" the body's engine are acids—pyruvic acid and lactic acid. These acids accumulate in the blood, muscles, and brain, with damaging effects. The cardiovascular, nervous, and gastrointestinal systems are also impaired. The body's whole "ignition-electrical system," the nervous system, can suffer adverse effects.

The "classic" syndrome of thiamine deficiency is *beriberi*. There are many forms of beriberi: dry beriberi, in which the principal lesions include muscular atrophy and inflammation of the nerve endings; wet beriberi, with general edema and internal effusions sometimes complicated with myocardial insufficiency; infantile beriberi; and a combination of wet and dry beriberi.

Thiamine deficiency also depresses protein synthesis in the brain and organs,[1] and depresses the uptake of two neurotransmitters, acetylcholine and serotonin, by the nerve synapses in the brain.[2] Without these chemicals, the transmission of nerve impulses is seriously impaired.

Thiamine deficiency also results in derangement of the appetite mechanisms, so that the sufferer loses the will to eat.[3] This effect is directly related to the inhibition of carbohydrate metabolism. When the "engine" is stalled, its desire for fuel necessarily dies right along with it.

Since the cells must operate at greatly reduced efficiency when the body's thiamine supply is inadequate, the production of cellular antibodies—an important part of the body's immune system—is severely diminished.[4]

The first symptom that thiamine demand exceeds supply is called *neurasthenia*, which is "doctorese" for nervous exhaustion. Appetite, memory, initiative, concentration, and temper are gradually lost right along with energy. They're replaced with fatigue and depression. Pains in the abdomen and chest follow. As the deficiency gets worse, "pins and needles" begin in the toes and burning sensations begin in the feet. What's happening is that the nerve pathways are degenerating. First the nerves go, then the muscles. The sense of touch seems to disappear, except that certain muscles in the legs start to feel very tender. Walking becomes more than a chore. And since the heart is a muscle, it starts to die, too.

The body prefers to take its energy supply, or fuel, in its natural state and refine it internally. So, if too much pure, high-octane fuel—sugar—is supplied, the engine/body eventually burns out—just as a car's engine would if supplied with over-refined gasoline. The most lethal form of highly refined sugar available to the body's engine is alcohol. Alcohol puts such great demands on the carbohydrate metabolism—fuel supply and ignition system—that it quickly burns up the enzyme systems involved. Thiamine is one of the first coenzymes to be used up when the body has to deal with too much alcohol. For this reason, alcoholics are susceptible to a special form of thiamine deficiency called *Wernicke-Korsakoff Syndrome*. The symptoms include: confusion, amnesia, palsy, loss of muscular coordination, paralysis of the eye muscles, involuntary jerking of the eyes, and coma.

All of the above hellish afflictions can be avoided or cured within hours by the administration of a few milligrams of thiamine—unless some metabolic defect is present which prevents the utilization of thiamine. Such a defect is present in *Leigh's Disease*. This genetic neurological disease involves a metabolic interference with the process by which thiamine is utilized by the nervous system.[5]

With the exception of alcoholics and people with Leigh's Disease, few people in developed countries are in danger of developing such a severe deficiency of thiamine. But let's not forget the continuum. A vast middle ground lies between getting enough thiamine and getting none or very little. That middle ground is populated by large numbers of people who may think their diets are adequate, but who nonetheless suffer lesser versions of many of the above symptoms. Naturally, we all suffer some of those symptoms from time to time. So every instance of fatigue, pins and needles, depression, or nervousness can't be blamed on thiamine deficiency. But chronic, persistent health problems can be caused by chronic, persistent weaknesses in the body's "ignition system."

Other Effects of Thiamine Deficiency

Thiamine is not usually thought of as a cause of anemia, yet doctors have reported at least one case of anemia that failed to respond to the conventional remedies but did respond to thiamine. The young woman who suffered the anemia apparently had a metabolic defect in a single enzyme that required thiamine. Dietary amounts of the vitamin weren't enough to overcome the defect, so supplementary doses were successfully employed.[6]

This case illustrates one of the things that can get in the way of a vitamin's doing its job. A person's requirement can be selectively raised in order to overcome a single defect in a single enzyme function which, as in the case of this young woman, doesn't happen to be one of the "classic" functions of the vitamin. Many people no doubt suffer such selective deficiencies until, by expert detective work or—as in the above case—by *accident*, the missing ingredient is supplied in a multivitamin pill.

Thiamine deficiency has been shown to cause eye problems, too. Two men, one a pilot and the other an aircraft mechanic, on low-carbohydrate, high-protein diets, suddenly had trouble seeing, especially when red light was the source of illumination. Tests revealed that their visual acuity was severely diminished to about 20/40 in both eyes. But after a few weeks on a regular diet, plus 50 mg. of thiamine daily, their vision was back to 20/20.[7]

CAN EXTRA THIAMINE DO US ANY GOOD?

Thiamine and Infection

Thiamine deficiency depresses the immune response, but does *extra* thiamine *stimulate* it? Apparently it does, because rabbits injected with thiamine before inoculation with tetanus toxin demonstrate more resistance to the toxin than animals which don't get extra thiamine. Not only does the thiamine keep the animals alive while other animals are killed by the toxin, but it also delays the spread of the disease.[8]

Thiamine and Multiple Sclerosis

Thiamine is an essential component of the myelin sheath, the "insulation" which is wrapped around the nerve fibers of the body. To use the car metaphor again, disintegration of the myelin sheath causes the same kind of problems that disintegration of the insulation on the wires in an automobile would cause: short circuits, scrambling of electrical signals, disabling of the mechanisms dependent upon electrical stimulation.

Canadian doctors attempted to find out if large doses of thiamine could affect the degeneration of the myelin sheath that occurs in multiple sclerosis. They injected 150 mg. of thiamine plus liver extract every week to ten days, and observed that while the treatments were continued, symptoms of the disease went away. When the treatment was stopped, or when *oral* thiamine was substituted, the symptoms returned. At the time this was reported (1973), some patients were still returning for the apparently successful treatment after twenty-nine years. The Canadian doctors don't claim they've found a cure for multiple sclerosis, but they do faithfully report what they've seen and done. They theorize that because the patients relapsed when oral thiamine was substituted for the injections, the people who were helped might not absorb thiamine through the digestive tract.[9]

In light of this research, it's difficult to rule out the possibility that a selective metabolic deficiency of thiamine plays a role in multiple sclerosis. For the people who have been helped by this treatment, it's a very important role, to say the least.

Thiamine and Cancer

Many researchers have reported that cancer patients have biochemical evidence of thiamine deficiency, even though they are not malnourished. Apparently the deficiency is caused by internal factors. An increase in the effectiveness of antitumor drugs when given with thiamine has been reported, too. These studies don't imply that cancer is caused by a thiamine deficiency, but rather that cancer patients may require more thiamine to fight off the disease.

Thiamine and Children

Thiamine is important to children for many reasons. Supplemental thiamine may be of help in stuttering. Many years ago a speech therapist instructed a pediatrician to give preschool children who stuttered moderate supplements of thiamine (25–30 mg. daily). The two- and three-year-olds were the most responsive: eighty percent of them improved. Half of the four-year-olds improved. None of the older children was helped. All who improved did so within two to three weeks of beginning the treatment. The doctors explain the treatment's success as a result of thiamine's effect on the nervous system.[10]

Thiamine deficiency can have profound and lasting effects on the nervous system of children. Animal experiments have shown that thiamine deficiency impairs learning, and that the defect persists even after the deficiency is corrected.[11]

An even more profound effect of thiamine deficiency has been theorized by a pediatrician at the Cleveland Clinic, Dr. Derrick Lonsdale. Dr. Lonsdale believes that the dread Sudden Infant Death Syndrome (SIDS) may be a result of an inborn metabolic defect in thiamine metabolism. This renders the nervous system of the infant unequal to the task of keeping the breathing process going. Dr. Lonsdale associates SIDS with infantile beriberi, and notes a mysterious *decline* in infant mortality from SIDS during wartime Hong Kong. It seems that when the Japanese occupied Hong Kong, they severely cut back the rice ration. After that, the SIDS death rate—which had been extremely high before the occupation—dropped to practically zero. When the occupation ended and the rice was restored, the SIDS rate skyrocketed again.

Dr. Lonsdale believes that the high carbohydrate, white rice diet exacerbated the effects of an inborn thiamine defect and caused the infants' deaths. But when the high carbohydrate diet was reduced, less of a burden was placed on the body's ability to utilize thiamine and keep the nervous system going.

The end product of Dr. Lonsdale's theory is his treatment of a number of babies with the symptoms of SIDS (the baby must have stopped breathing on at least one occasion). Using supplements of 30–300 mg. of thiamine per day, Dr. Lonsdale has seen the SIDS symptoms disappear in all the infants he has treated.[12]

Thiamine has a role in cases where an *adult's* nervous system goes awry, too. Thiamine levels were measured in 65 neurotic patients and found low. The researchers speculate that the increasing numbers of neurotic persons could be a result of low-level thiamine deficiency caused by the overconsumption of refined foods low in thiamine.[13] (I don't know if forgetful rats are considered neurotic, but Japanese researchers found they could improve the memory of rats merely by giving them a diet rich in thiamine. Depriving them of thiamine made their memories worse.[14])

HOW MUCH THIAMINE DO WE NEED?

Beriberi has existed for thousands of years, but up until the last half of the nineteenth century, it was a disease primarily of the rich. We usually don't think of rich people as suffering from nutritional deficiencies, but many of the B vitamin deficiencies were suffered by the upper classes for centuries before they were "handed down" to the poor. The reason for this is that only the rich could afford refined food such as white rice and flour—up until the nineteenth century, when milling of grain became widespread and inexpensive. So when millions of people began to depend on polished rice, which is practically devoid of thiamine, instead of brown rice, beriberi became a disease of the masses.

The body's requirement for thiamine is dependent upon two factors: the caloric content of the diet, especially with regard to carbohydrates, and the amount of energy expended. So someone eating a high carbohydrate diet and using a lot of energy needs more thiamine than someone who eats very little carbohydrate and sits still all day. Of course, there is a bottom-line requirement for thiamine, which even the sedentary person who doesn't eat much has to fulfill. That baseline, the RDA, is 1 mg. (Actually, the RDA is set at .5 mg. for every 1000 calories in the daily diet.)

But many factors can enter the picture and raise that requirement. Pregnant and lactating women need more thiamine. Alcoholics are at great risk for thiamine deficiency.

Alcohol metabolizes as a carbohydrate, so it burns up B vitamins but doesn't replace them. An equal caloric load of whole grains, for example, would resupply much if not all of the thiamine which was required to metabolize it.

Fever, hyperthyroidism, liver disorders, and diseases which interfere with digestion and metabolism can also raise thiamine requirements. You can get a thiamine deficiency in the hospital from the heavy carbohydrate load of the intravenous feeding.[15] Food high in tannin, or tannic acid, can cause a thiamine deficiency. Tannin, which is high in tea and betel nuts, destroys thiamine in the body. Vitamin C partially inhibits and reverses the destruction, however.[16] In one study, human volunteers drinking tea along with a normal diet exhibited both biochemical and clinical symptoms of thiamine deficiency.[17] A quart of tea destroys about twice the RDA of thiamine.[18] Coffee also destroys thiamine in the body. A quart of coffee consumed over a three-hour period was shown to destroy most of the body's store of thiamine. (The villain in coffee is not tannin, or even caffeine, but chlorogenic acid.[19])

Women using oral contraceptives are in danger of a thiamine deficiency, too. In one study, at least 3 mg. daily of extra thiamine was necessary to make up for the deficiency caused by the oral contraceptives.[20]

Who else needs more thiamine? People who are deficient in other B vitamins, such as pyridoxine (B6) and cobalamin (B12), certainly do, because deficiencies in these two vitamins interfere with thiamine metabolism.[21]

Older women may need more thiamine, too, just to maintain adequate levels in their bodies. Older women have been shown to excrete less thiamine than younger women on similar diets. The implication of this is that the older women were *using* more than the younger women, or at least they needed more thiamine to maintain adequate levels of vitamin activity in their bodies. When the women were placed on thiamine-deficient diets for a while, and then put back on adequate diets, the older women took longer to recover from the effects of the deficiency.[22]

Athletes, because they consume and expend more energy, obviously would be a risk for a thiamine deficiency. Such deficiencies have been reported.[23]

People with chronic liver disease, both alcoholics and nonalcoholics, have been reported deficient in thiamine, and should receive more than the RDA.[24]

What do all these factors add up to? Researchers have reported that up to twenty percent of the population of *developed* countries such as the United States, Canada, and Great Britain, have "below adequate" thiamine status. And that *half* of the people in developing countries are deficient.[25] One study, however, found that *seventy-five percent* of surveyed Home Economics majors were not meeting the RDA for thiamine in their diets. They were not alcoholics, athletes, or any of the other groups that risk thiamine deficiency. In fact, they were the last group of people you'd expect to not be getting enough vitamins from their food.[26] So if a Home Economics expert ever tells you that you can get all the vitamins you need from your diet alone, think twice.

SOURCES OF THIAMINE

Thiamine is available in supplemental form in a wide range of dosages, from 1 mg. all the way up to hundreds of milligrams. Thiamine is nontoxic, and allergic intolerance is rare. Doses as high as 500 mg. per day have been given for periods up to a month with no signs of toxicity.[27]

The richest natural sources of thiamine are organ meats such as liver, heart, and kidney. Yeast, lean meat, eggs, green leafy vegetables, whole grain cereals, nuts, berries, and legumes are also good sources. White rice and flour have been rendered void of thiamine by processing, but small amounts are "fortified" back. Thiamine is water-soluble and destroyed by oxidation. Cooking in water contributes to thiamine loss when the vitamin dissolves in the water and becomes vulnerable to oxidation.

3

Riboflavin (B₂)

If thiamine is the spark plug of the body's engine, riboflavin is the carburetor. Besides fuel and a spark to ignite the fuel, an engine needs to *breathe*. Riboflavin is one of the B vitamins that's essential for cellular respiration. So without riboflavin, the cells don't breathe and the body's engine suffocates.

Your car may be brand new with a gleaming new coat of wax and an engine tuned to race, but if you inhibit the flow of air to the cylinders, it probably won't even start. The same is true for the body's engine. And if you do manage to get started, you'll certainly be in no condition to race.

Riboflavin is also involved in the metabolism of vitamin C, because when experimental animals are maintained on a riboflavin-deficient diet, some of their first symptoms resemble those of vitamin C deficiency.[1] A riboflavin deficiency can also lead to a deficiency of other B vitamins which depend on it for their metabolism. Pyridoxine is especially susceptible.[2]

WHAT HAPPENS WHEN RIBOFLAVIN DEMAND
EXCEEDS SUPPLY

If a rag blew into your car's air scoop and reduced the amount of air available to the engine, unless you were trained to distinguish the symptoms, you might think every nut and bolt in the engine was loose and every gasket and seal leaking. Likewise, if the cells' respiration is impeded, the symptoms can make you feel as if you need a major overhaul. Growth failure, weight loss, disturbances in the structure and function of the eyes, adrenal glands, nerves, skin, and mucous membranes have all been attributed to riboflavin deficiency.

Riboflavin deficiency has profound effects on the metabolism of carbohydrates, fats, and protein. All three of these basic food elements require riboflavin if they are to be properly utilized by the body. When not enough riboflavin is supplied, carbohydrate utilization decreases, so the body "tells" itself to consume more carbohydrates to make up for the diminished efficiency.

When the vitamin is undersupplied, protein utilization also drops off. More protein is excreted in the urine. This begins a vicious cycle, because when more protein has to be excreted, the increased urinary output will also eliminate *more riboflavin* from the body. (Remember, any factor that increases excretion—urine, sweat, feces—also increases the loss of water-soluble vitamins.)

Dietary fat also increases the body's need for riboflavin. When insufficient riboflavin is supplied to handle the fat in the diet, the fat is deposited in the liver, kidneys, adrenals, and arterial walls.[3]

Naturally, such interference with the metabolism of the three basic food elements will have profound effects on energy production and tissue structure. For example, the adrenal glands of riboflavin-deficient animals and people become exhausted and eventually atrophy. This results in a drop in the output of adrenal hormones and a severe decrease in the formation of red blood cells.[4] Both of these effects are going to mean an "engine" that's not going to want to get off the starting line, let alone race.

Riboflavin deficiency also interferes with the activity of the thyroid gland, and produces birth defects which affect the nervous system, skin, skeleton, and vascular system.[5] In young animals, riboflavin deficiency diminishes learning capacity. Such effects apparently linger, because supplying adequate riboflavin when the animals are older does not restore normal learning.[6]

HOW DO YOU KNOW IF YOU'RE GETTING ENOUGH RIBOFLAVIN?

As with all other vitamins and minerals, you won't necessarily suffer the "classic" symptoms of a deficiency. A person whose riboflavin demands exceed the supply *may* have an inflamed tongue, lips, or mouth. The eyes can become oversensitive to light and will itch, burn, and appear bloodshot and teary. Seborrheic (greasy scaling) dermatitis will afflict the area around the lips and nose, eyes, behind the ears, and scrotum. Any of these symptoms can be caused by many other factors. However, if they all appear together and a person's diet is suspect, the finger of suspicion points to riboflavin deficiency.

The changes which occur in the eyes may be especially important. Riboflavin deficiency produces opacities in the eyes of animals identical to those caused by cataracts.[7] Corneal opacity has also been found in people with riboflavin deficiency. And when doctors tested twenty-two people with cataracts, they found that eight of them had cellular deficiencies of riboflavin.[8]

Riboflavin deficiency can produce psychiatric disturbances, too. In one riboflavin-deficiency study, six young men were maintained on a riboflavin-deficient diet—under twenty-four-hour medical supervision—and given batteries of psychological tests. Significant psychological changes took place as the deficiencies took hold. The men felt more lethargic and depressed. They complained more about pains and illnesses they didn't have (hypochondriasis). They scored higher on hysteria and psychopathic-deviate scales, and underwent measurable personality shifts. Interestingly, none of the "classic" symptoms of riboflavin deficiency (dermatitis, inflammation of the eyes, etc.) appeared before the experiment ended. And when the men were given riboflavin at the end of the experiment—some two months or more after it began—it took more than two weeks for all of the psychiatric symptoms to disappear.[9]

In another study of the psychological effects of vitamins, researchers associated high blood levels of riboflavin with increased extroversion, concentration, and contentment.[10]

The former study seems to suggest that we can suffer debilitating effects of a riboflavin deficiency *before* the standard, medically recognized symptoms appear. Here again, remember the continuum. We can only speculate on how many people have psychological problems which might respond to riboflavin.

Therapeutic Uses of Riboflavin

Swiss doctors discovered that adding 3 mg. of riboflavin to an iron supplement given to anemic pregnant women increased the effectiveness and durability of the treatment.[11]

Riboflavin may have a beneficial effect upon the *muscles' ability to perform*. Giving young athletes a moderate riboflavin supplement has been reported to increase their resistance to fatigue by about eleven percent. In a separate experiment, young athletes were given 10 mg. of riboflavin, and their neuromuscular irritability—a biochemical measurement associated with fatigue—was lowered. Eight of the athletes were deficient in riboflavin, however, before the supplementation. This not only suggests an increased need for riboflavin during training and exercise, but also that a riboflavin supplement might be a good idea for athletes. Especially athletes who have to perform in the cold, since animal experiments have demonstrated that riboflavin in high doses enabled rats to swim for longer periods in cold water.[12]

Riboflavin apparently helps *protect the body* by maintaining the immune response and by detoxifying noxious chemicals that enter the body. Cellular antibody production and activity is diminished in riboflavin deficiency.[13] Riboflavin also helps the liver detoxify chemicals such as estrogens, carcinogens, and other harmful natural and synthetic chemicals.[14] The discovery that boric acid poisoning causes excessive levels of riboflavin in the urine led doctors to speculate that the vitamin may be involved in detoxifying the common poison.[15]

As mentioned, riboflavin detoxifies cancer-causing chemicals. In one experiment, riboflavin prevented the formation of liver tumors in rats treated with such chemicals. Riboflavin deficiency has been shown to stimulate growth of tumors. Less riboflavin than normal is excreted in cases of cancer of the stomach, breast, uterus, skin, and lung—an indication of increased utilization and need.[16] In one study of 1000 adults with cancer, virtually *no* riboflavin was excreted by eighty percent of the people, regardless of where the tumor was.[17]

Once again, none of the researchers responsible for these findings would suggest that cancer is a result of riboflavin deficiency. What their findings imply, however, is that riboflavin deficiency may indeed be a factor in the progression of the disease. Obviously, riboflavin plays an important role in the body's defenses against cancer, as do many other nutrients.

HOW MUCH RIBOFLAVIN DO WE NEED?

The RDA for riboflavin varies according to weight, metabolic rate, growth, and caloric intake, and ranges from .4 mg. for infants to 1.9 mg. for lactating women, with male adults requiring 1.7 mg. and female adults 1.2 mg. Remember, the RDA is an arbitrary figure and does not necessarily bear any relation to what an individual's needs really might be. Some researchers recommend higher dietary amounts, with supplementation during periods of stress or exertion.

Nonetheless, how do we stand on riboflavin? Not as well as we should, apparently. Dietary riboflavin levels fall short of requirements in one out of seven families in the USA[18], and from ten to twenty percent of minorities in the USA are deficient.[19] One study measured riboflavin status (biochemical, not dietary) in diabetic and normal children and found twenty-six percent of the diabetic children and almost nine percent of the normal children deficient. All the children were given riboflavin supplements and their deficiencies went away.[20] Riboflavin deficiency appears to be prevalent among children suffering from heart disease. In one study, thirty-five percent of children measured had biochemical evidence of deficiency. Among the riboflavin deficient children, there was a greater frequency of congestive heart failure.[21]

What are some of the factors causing riboflavin deficiency? A high fat diet can boost riboflavin requirements. And a protein deficiency, by causing increased excretion, also causes more riboflavin to be lost.

There are some particular "stresses" that can cause a riboflavin deficiency, too. Riboflavin is destroyed by light. Doctors have found that phototherapy of newborn infants for the treatment of jaundice also causes a riboflavin deficiency. They believe this effect may be responsible for the "failure to thrive" syndrome these infants often suffer.[22]

There are other "iatrogenic" (caused by doctors) riboflavin deficiencies. Malnutrition often occurs in hospital patients, and one of the distinct features of protein-calorie malnutrition is riboflavin deficiency.

Oral contraceptives raise riboflavin requirements, because these chemicals (estrogens) must be detoxified in the liver, and any liver detoxification process requires riboflavin and other B vitamins. There are numerous reports of this phenomenon. In one study, half of the women on the Pill and eleven percent of those not on the Pill were deficient. Of the women who had been on the Pill for three or more years, eighty-two percent were deficient.[23] One study found that it took riboflavin supplements of 2 mg. per day to overcome oral contraceptive-induced riboflavin deficiency.[24]

Riboflavin deficiency can be caused by other drugs, such as phenothiazines (tranquilizers)[25] and antibiotics.[26]

SOURCES OF RIBOFLAVIN

The richest natural sources of riboflavin include organ meats, fish, dairy products, eggs, green leafy vegetables, wheat germ, whole grains, and legumes. Riboflavin is not destroyed by heat, but soaking foods or cooking them in water for long periods of time can result in substantial losses, since the vitamin is water-soluble. Exposure to light will also destroy riboflavin.

Riboflavin is available in a wide range of supplementary dosages, from less than 1 mg. to hundreds of milligrams. Riboflavin is not toxic. Attempts to produce toxic reactions in experimental animals failed.[27] Taking riboflavin along with food or fiber increases absorption of the vitamin.[28]

4

Niacin (B₃)

Of all the B vitamins, niacin is undoubtedly the most controversial. Hundreds of physicians and nutritionists use niacin to treat three of the most persistently damaging diseases of our time: heart disease, mental illness, and arthritis.

WHAT NIACIN DOES

Niacin's basic function is to assist in cellular respiration and in the cell's utilization of all major nutrients. The two co-enzymes which require niacin have been identified as necessary to at least *forty* different biochemical reactions. Without question, niacin is one of the most important factors in keeping us moving toward the optimum health end of the continuum.

Niacin is a mild vasodilator, which means that it widens the diameter of blood vessels and increases blood flow. High doses of niacin lower high blood cholesterol and cause a reaction called the "niacin flush," in which the skin temperature increases, the face reddens, and the blood pressure temporarily drops. Dizziness may occur, too.

High doses of niacin also inhibit the mobilization of fat from the tissues. This effect has implications for alcoholics, dieters, athletes, and people with heart disease. Alcohol has the opposite effect: it mobilizes fat from the tissues and much of that increased blood fat ends up in the liver. In the livers of test animals, extremely high doses of niacin can prevent this accumulation of fat.[1] While niacin undoubtedly has a protective effect on the liver, as many B vitamins do, the doses used in this particular experiment were too high to have immediate practical implications. If you need such high doses of niacin to protect your liver from alcohol, you're consuming too much alcohol. Besides, the niacin in this experiment also served to keep alcohol in the blood longer. So, ultimately, the liver protection may be a bad bargain if other organs are exposed to alcohol for a longer period.

High doses of niacin (actually niacin*amide*, a different form of niacin about which more later) were also found to increase the amount of rapid eye movement sleep (REM sleep is the most restful level of sleep) in animals. Again, however, the doses were so high this effect has little relevance to the sleeping problems of normal people. Such an effect, however, may have implications in the treatment of mentally ill persons.[2]

WHAT HAPPENS WHEN
NIACIN DEMAND EXCEEDS SUPPLY

The classic deficiency syndrome of niacin is called *pellagra*. Because of niacin's crucial role in the most basic biochemical reactions, every cell in the body can be affected by a deficiency. The three major "target" organs of pellagra are the skin, the gastrointestinal tract, and the nervous system. There is some evidence that a prolonged deficiency of niacin can result in a more or less permanent "dependency," or increased requirement, for the vitamin.[3]

The best-known symptoms of niacin deficiency, or pellagra, are the "3-Ds:" dermatitis, diarrhea, and dementia. The dermatitis in part resembles that of other B vitamin deficiencies, with swollen, bluish tongue, and inflamed mouth and lips. But these are the least of the manifestations on the skin. The skin may become red, blistery, infected, fissured, scaly, or hardened. These lesions usually appear on areas of the body exposed to sunlight or trauma. Elbows and knees, the backs of the neck and hands, and the forearms are common areas afflicted. The mucous membranes of the mouth may become sore and ulcerated and eventually hemorrhage.

The mucous membranes of the gastrointestinal tract are similarly affected. Digestive secretions are diminished, and burning, gastric discomfort, distention, flatulence, and occasional vomiting give way to severe diarrhea.

A comparable disaster takes place in the nervous system. The first symptoms are mild anxiety, apprehension, fatigue, loss of appetite, skin hypersensitivity, digestive upset, headache, insomnia, tension, and alternating depression and hyperactivity. These progress to irritability, emotional instability, and various psychotic symptoms such as hallucinations, confusion, disorientation, paranoia, delirium, mania, failing vision, hypersensitivity to light, hyperacute sense of smell, dulled sense of taste, and severe depression.

There is a group of symptoms sometimes found in niacin deficiency distinct from pellagra. Some of the less severe manifestations of dermatitis may be present, along with clouding of consciousness, "cogwheel" rigidity of the extremities, uncontrollable grasping and sucking reflexes, and coma. This syndrome generally appears in hospitalized people who have been maintained on intravenous feeding without vitamin supplementation for long periods of time.

Once these deficiencies have taken hold, it requires doses of niacin many times the usual amount in order to treat them successfully. If they have been longstanding deficiencies, the damage to the nervous system may not always be completely reparable. And the subject may need higher doses of niacin permanently in order to keep the deficiency from returning.

Niacin and Mental Illness

Considering the effect of niacin deficiency on the nervous system, it's difficult to understand how anyone could seriously doubt that niacin metabolism plays *some* role in mental illness. Yet niacin's role is one of the most heated controversies in psychiatry.

The doctors who believe niacin has some benefit in the treatment of mental illness are known as "orthomolecular" psychiatrists or physicians. *Orthomolecular* refers to the basis of their treatment, which is to use chemicals normally found in the body to correct molecular balances which have gone awry in critical functions. This, of course, is directly opposite to the basis of most modern medicine, which uses drugs— chemicals which are foreign to the body—and surgery, to *interfere* with normal body processes. You can immediately understand why both sides might have difficulty acknowledging the other: You couldn't have two more opposing views of therapeutics!

Since this is a book about vitamins and minerals, let's continue describing niacin's role in mental health, without giving any more deference to the "other side" than common sense dictates. No doctor who uses niacin to treat mental illness claims it is beneficial in all cases.

Nonetheless, it does seem to be of use in *some* cases. There are so many reports by sincere, dedicated, skillful physicians and psychiatrists of schizophrenia cases greatly improved after niacin therapy that it would be impossible to write that there really is a question of whether niacin is of use in mental illness.[4] Some studies have shown that it makes about the same number of patients worse as it does better.[5] This is no reason to discount its usefulness. Many current conventional therapies have no better track records.

Canadian physician Abram Hoffer is one of the principal champions of orthomolecular medicine. Dr. Hoffer reported his experience with more than twenty years' use of niacin in the treatment of schizophrenia: seventy-five percent of his patients who received niacin therapy (3 grams per day, on average) did not require hospitalization, whereas only thirty-six percent of those receiving conventional therapies did not require hospitalization.[6] Dr. Hoffer also reported the use of niacin to restore mental health to a young woman who had been mildly ill since childhood. At the age of twelve the girl was diagnosed as having degenerative disease of the spinal cord and brain, and schizophrenia. When her psychotic symptoms worsened, she was placed on tranquilizers—with only slight improvement. Dr. Hoffer examined the girl when she was fifteen and quickly placed her on niacin therapy. Her improvement was steady and permanent. Her mental health was apparently restored, since at the time of the report she was finishing school and getting married. Dr. Hoffer concluded that she was suffering from niacin-dependent schizophrenia, but that there had been no permament deterioration of her brain or spinal cord.[7]

One researcher attempted to find out if certain types of schizophrenia were more likely to respond to niacin therapy. He found that those who had a healthy personality history before the onset of their acute illness, with "strong interpersonal commitments," were more likely to respond to niacin therapy.[8] Other studies have shown niacin to be of use in treating obsessive-compulsive behavior,[9] and to potentiate the therapeutic effects of phenothiazine drugs given to schizophrenia patients.[10]

I think it's important to point out that the dosages used in these treatments are extremely high, and are not given without careful observation. Orthomolecular physicians seldom administer "megadoses" of vitamins without taking into consideration the results of various biomedical tests which indicate certain enzyme levels in the body. Their aim is to correct enzymatic defects that cause the disease.

The implications for those of us who are not mentally ill

are that perhaps some of our day-to-day mental lapses might have something to do with the state of our nutrition.

Niacin and Heart Disease

Because niacin dilates the blood vessels, temporarily lowers blood pressure, and appears to lower blood cholesterol, there is a certain amount of controversy surrounding its use as a treatment in heart disease. The primary problem in heart disease is the blockage of blood vessels. Any factor which widens the blood vessels and restores circulation is of possible benefit. High blood pressure and blood cholesterol also appear to heighten the risk of developing heart disease. So any factor which can lower blood pressure and/or cholesterol levels is a potential aid, too.

So, in theory at least, niacin looks as if it might be helpful for those with heart disease. Pellagra victims often have abnormal electrocardiograms, which are an indication of abnormal heart function. The abnormalities disappear when the deficiency is treated.[11]

The National Heart, Lung, and Blood Institute performed a massive eight-year study involving over 8000 heart patients, over 1000 of whom were given niacin therapy. Niacin appeared to have no better effect than dummy pills, or "placebo" treatments. Cholesterol *was* definitely lowered, but this lowering had no effect with regard to keeping the patients alive longer than any other patients. The only significant effect seemed to be that niacin-treated patients experienced fewer nonfatal heart attacks over the five-year duration of their treatment.[12] Since niacin did no worse, and in some cases better, than other drugs used to lower cholesterol, it's still considered a useful "drug" for lowering cholesterol.

It's important to point out that niacin is in no way the single answer to heart disease. Simply lowering blood levels of cholesterol is not enough. Even if it *were*, to believe that a single agent—whether a vitamin or a drug—could make up for the damaging effects of a high-fat, high-sugar diet, and a lifestyle that considers walking to the car a form of exercise, is folly. Heart disease is not caused by a deficiency of niacin, and no matter how much niacin you take, there are other things that you should do if you really want to avoid the disease that kills more Americans than does anything else.

Niacin and Arthritis

Dr. William Kaufman began using niacin more than thirty years ago to treat many of the symptoms we commonly associate with aging. Dr. Kaufman observed that many of his patients complained of ailments that were similar to the symptoms of niacin deficiency: fatigue, gastrointestinal upset, skin problems, confusion, and irritability. In addition, many of them had joints that were stiffening more and more each day, making life difficult and painful.

Dr. Kaufman knew these people did not have classic cases of pellagra. But he was aware of that continuum of effects of vitamin deficiencies. Wasn't it possible, he theorized, that these people were suffering from *mild* cases of pellagra? He tried giving them niacin (actually, he used the niacinamide form). Much to his surprise, many of their symptoms vanished. Most people came back reporting great improvement.

Dr. Kaufman started keeping elaborate records of his patients' progress. He devised tools to measure their joint flexibility and strength and made more recordings of progress. Over the next thirty years of his practice (he is now retired), he helped hundreds and hundreds of people regain joint flexibility they thought they had lost for good. He used niacinamide in doses of from 900 mg. to 4000 mg. per day. Dr. Kaufman published a book and many papers about his work.[13]

Skepticism cannot take Dr. Kaufman's achievements away from him, or from the many people he helped. Other doctors use Dr. Kaufman's method of treating joint stiffness, and are sharing his success.

HOW MUCH NIACIN DO WE NEED?

The RDA for niacin varies from 6 mg. for babies to 13 mg. for adult women and 18 mg. for men and lactating women. Many times these amounts are usually required to overcome the effects of a deficiency, since one of the lingering effects is diminished gastrointestinal function. The mentally ill people who respond to niacin therapy in the megadose range most likely have metabolic deficiencies caused by defects in certain enzyme systems which require niacin. The large doses of niacin, in effect, *force* the enzyme reactions to function.

The same cannot be said for niacin's use in heart disease. This is a "pharmaceutical" or "drug" effect, in which large doses of the vitamin force a reaction to take place which may be desirable but which does not normally occur. The amounts of niacin used in both these treatments run into the thousands of milligrams.

What about the rest of us who do not have heart disease, schizophrenia, nor arthritis? Are we getting enough niacin in our diets?

The story of pellagra illustrates one of the clearest pictures of how devastating a nutritional "fad" can be. When corn was introduced to Europe from the New World, it eventually became a major staple of the diet of countries around the Mediterranean Sea. As corn flourished, so did pellagra. Why? Because corn replaced other foods that supplied *tryptophan*, an essential element of protein. The body can synthesize niacin from tryptophan. Corn supplies very little tryptophan; hence, pellagra. The same thing happened in the United States at the turn of the twentieth century, when farmers started growing corn by the millions of bushels. Not only wards of hospitals, but *entire mental hospitals* were set up to care for pellagrins.

People did not want to believe that pellagra was a result of poor nutrition. They insisted it was an infection of some sort. (At that time, the germ theory of disease was at its zenith.) So the bacteriologist who traced the disease to poor nutrition had to prove his case by eating and inoculating himself, his wife, and colleagues with biological specimens and excreta from known pellagrins. He proved his point,[14] but the hard way.

What the Europeans and Americans didn't know, and should have known before they made corn a dietary staple, was that the New World Indians who "lived on" corn mixed it and processed it with various alkaline ingredients which made tryptophan more readily available and averted a niacin deficiency. There's a lesson here for people who would exclusively adopt certain foodstuffs on which people in different cultures seem to thrive. Now that we have lost our dietary innocence and have a wide variety of foods in our reach, we should make the most of that opportunity.

Pellagra is not as uncommon as we might like to think. A group of doctors from Johns Hopkins University and Case Western Reserve University—certainly not bastions of radical nutritionism—found that "pellagra is a serious, not uncommon, and initially undiagnosed complication of malnutrition in today's urban society." These doctors also found that fewer that thirty percent of the pellagrins actually presented all of the classic symptoms.[15]

Niacin deficiency is usually found in people with chronically bad dietary habits; people who consume low-calorie, low-protein, high fat and carbohydrate diets; alcoholics; and people with diseases that interfere with digestion and absorption (these include chronic diarrhea, cirrhosis of the liver, and tuberculosis). Since pyridoxine (vitamin B_6) is necessary for the conversion of tryptophan to niacin, people with a deficiency in that vitamin may also have a deficiency in niacin. *Hartnup's Disease* is an inherited defect in tryptophan-niacin metabolism which produces an increased requirement for niacin in order to prevent the symptoms of pellagra.[16]

IS NIACIN TOXIC?

The niacin flush is not harmful, although it may be unsettling. The flush comes on within ten minutes and lasts about a half hour. The super high doses used by doctors treating heart disease and mental illness have caused minor side effects: nausea and itching. Doctors have reported that niacin in high doses should not be given to people with peptic ulcers, high blood pressure, diabetes, gout, or liver disease.[17]

SOURCES OF NIACIN

Rich natural sources of niacin include organ meats, fish, yeast, whole grains, dried peas and beans, and nuts. Corn *contains* tryptophan, from which the body can synthesize niacin, but the tryptophan is "bound" and cannot be used. Treating the corn with alkali releases the tryptophan for use. (This is the process the Indians of North America learned and the Europeans didn't.) Niacin is soluble in hot water, so cooking foods by boiling may result in substantial losses.

There are two forms of niacin: niacinamide and nicotinic acid (usually referred to simply as niacin). Niacin comes from plants, niacinamide from animals. In the human body, niacin is rapidly converted to niacinamide. Niacinamide is identical to niacin in all respects and functions except that it does not cause vasodilation or the niacin flush.

Niacin and niacinamide are available in a wide range of supplemental doses, from a few milligrams to 1000 milligrams.

An attempt to find out the "ideal" niacin intake, similar to the study described in the vitamin A chapter, found that health complaints and disease symptoms were fewest at a daily intake of 115 mg.[18] This study shouldn't be taken too literally. Any attempt to set the "ideal" or "adequate" daily requirement of any nutrient contradicts what we know of the wide variation in natural processes. This study does suggest, however, that the RDA for niacin may be too low.

5

Pyridoxine (B₆)

Pyridoxine could very easily become known as the "woman's vitamin," because it can help alleviate so many of the health problems peculiar to women, such as menstrual irregularities, premenstrual tension and acne, Pill-associated depression, complications of pregnancy, and many others.

It could just as easily become known as the "man's vitamin" because of its reported role in the prevention of heart disease.

And, of course, it could also come to be known as the "children's vitamin," because of its role in preventing birth defects, aiding the treatment of childhood mental illness, and curing convulsive disorders of infancy.

For all of the above reasons, plus its application in arthritis, diabetes, and detoxification, pyridoxine should simply be called the "people's vitamin." Certainly it's one of the most important factors in keeping us as close as possible to the optimum health end of the continuum.

Pyridoxine first became a household word back in the early 1950s, when a strange malady began attacking hundreds of newborn babies. All over the country, infants from two to four months old started scaring their parents to death by going into generalized *convulsions* several times a day. Otherwise, the children were perfectly healthy. And the families were not poor. All of them could afford to feed their babies manufactured infant formula.

Most of the babies were brought to the hospital by their anxious parents, where, as mysteriously as the convulsions had appeared, they disappeared. Medical sleuthing detected that all the infants had been fed one particular brand of infant formula, SMA. When they were changed to another formula or evaporated milk, they became free of convulsions. Something in the formula? No, something *not* in the formula: pyridoxine. Wyeth Laboratories, manufacturers of SMA, had somehow managed to produce pyridoxine-free formula.

Besides pointing out one of the many effects of a pyridoxine deficiency, this incident demonstrates the hazards of relying on man-made food, especially when a superior natural food—breast milk in this case—is readily available.

WHAT PYRIDOXINE DOES

Pyridoxine is an essential coenzyme for many, if not all, of the biochemical reactions involving amino acids, the individual substances that make up protein. These amino acids must be broken down, digested, absorbed, interconverted, and then taken up by the cells. Pyridoxine is required for all of these things to happen. One example is the requirement for pyridoxine in the conversion of the amino acid tryptophan to niacin.

Pyridoxine also plays an important role in the body's metabolism of fats and carbohydrates. The synthesis of unsaturated fatty acids requires pyridoxine. Energy cannot be produced for the cells without the vitamin.

WHAT HAPPENS WHEN PYRIDOXINE DEMAND
EXCEEDS SUPPLY

Because amino acids are the basic "building blocks" of all living tissue, and because they are constantly needed all over the body for repair and growth as well as the production of energy, a deficiency of pyridoxine can do widespread damage.

One of the first systems to suffer the effects of a deficiency is the nervous system. These effects are more pronounced and lingering in developing children and animals. The convulsions suffered by the infants fed pyridoxine-free formula would eventually have progressed to permanent mental retardation, or even death, had they persisted. The brain needs protein for development and function, and in a pyridoxine deficiency, the protein supply to the brain is severely curtailed.[1]

A deficiency of pyridoxine interferes with the development of the entire organism, not only the brain. When pregnant animals are maintained on diets containing various levels of pyridoxine, the offspring of the deficient groups are small, sickly, and have impaired motor development. Interestingly, the animals whose mothers are fed diets containing four times the "required" or "adequate" amount of pyridoxine are substantially healthier and better developed than those fed the standard amount.[2]

Pyridoxine deficiency not only interferes with the metabolism of the building blocks of life, but also with the *cement* that holds the building blocks together: collagen.[3] Such a defect can have adverse effects on the structural integrity of just about *any* part of the body. For example, the teeth can become stunted, deformed, demineralized, soft, decayed, and misaligned. The gums can become severely inflamed. Animals maintained on a diet with the same level of pyridoxine that occurs in the average American diet had more tooth decay than animals fed the same diet supplemented with extra pyridoxine. In another study, there was a forty percent reduction in tooth decay among children receiving a supplement of

9 mg. of pyridoxine a day, compared with children receiving a placebo supplement.[4]

Pyridoxine deficiency impairs the immune response. During pregnancy, this deficiency reduces the size of the thymus gland—which is involved in the immune response—in both mother and fetus. A deficiency of pyridoxine *before* pregnancy can also impair the newborn's capacity to fight off disease.[5]

Pyridoxine deficiency also impairs the function of the liver, and prolonged deficiency can cause permanent damage. Whether because of its role in liver function or its role in fat metabolism—probably both—a pyridoxine deficiency raises blood levels of cholesterol. In fact, animals maintained on such a deficiency, with one percent of their diet in cholesterol, will have higher-than-normal levels of cholesterol in their blood. Animals maintained on pyridoxine-deficient diets also develop arteriosclerosis.[6]

Common Deficiency Symptoms

The standardly recognized symptoms of pyridoxine deficiency include greasy, scaling dermatitis around the eyes, ears, nose, and mouth, and in areas that frequently rub together, such as the inner thighs. Inflammation of the oral area, identical to that which occurs in other B vitamin deficiencies, is also possible. The neuromuscular effects—convulsions, nerve tissue degeneration—can occur in adults and children.

Some people are born with a greatly increased need, or dependency, for pyridoxine. A fortunate few may be identified early enough to be treated and saved from mental retardation. Obviously, however, not all mental retardation is a result of pyridoxine deficiency.

Pyridoxine and Oral Contraceptives

Pyridoxine deficiency occurs in many women taking the Pill. In one study, women from upper socioeconomic groups, and on the Pill, had biochemical evidence of pyridoxine deficiency more often than women from lower socioeconomic groups and not on the Pill.[4]

The result of this pyridoxine deficiency is not convulsions, it's depression. Apparently, the deficiency interferes with the metabolism of certain amino acids in the brain. Not *all* women become depressed when using oral contraceptives. And of those who do, not *all* depression is necessarily due to pyridoxine deficiency. But among women on the Pill who also have a pyridoxine deficiency, the administration of pyridoxine supplements usually alleviates the depression.

Some doctors have attempted to predict which women will respond best to pyridoxine. From their research, they've concluded that women with a history of depression, premenstrual depression, or depression during pregnancy—and who become worse after starting the Pill—are most likely to respond to pyridoxine. In one study, 220 out of 250 such women responded to pyridoxine therapy for their depression. What about women who don't have a particular history of depression, and yet are depressed when they take oral contraceptives? If they have a pyridoxine deficiency, chances are they will respond to supplements. In a test of this, all of the women (about half of a group of depressed women on the Pill) who had the biochemical signs of a deficiency got well again with pyridoxine supplementation.[8] The dose of pyridoxine used to alleviate Pill-induced depression ranges from 25 mg. to over 100 mg. per day.

Another side effect of the Pill is a derangement of glucose tolerance-carbohydrate metabolism: the body's ability to utilize carbohydrates and clear sugar from the bloodstream can be severely impaired. In some women, this impairment can reach a state identical to diabetes.[9] In one study, although all of the women taking the Pill had evidence of abnormal tryptophan metabolism (a sign the Pill had impaired their pyridoxine metabolism), not all were affected enough to cause a pyridoxine deficiency. However, *all* the *deficient* women had impaired glucose tolerance, while none of the other women did.[10] In another study, it was shown that pyridoxine supplements of 25 mg. could restore glucose tolerance in these women.[11]

Pyridoxine and Pregnancy

The same impairment of carbohydrate metabolism that sometimes occurs as a side effect of the Pill also happens to some pregnant women. When it does, it's called "gestational diabetes." Pyridoxine deficiency is usually present. In one study, fourteen women with gestational diabetes were given 100 mg. of pyridoxine each day. Within two weeks, the glucose tolerance of twelve of the women was normal again.[12] Apparently many pregnant women undergo at least a slight impairment of glucose tolerance. In some, the effects of this can be deadly for both mother and child. Many of the researchers who carry out these studies on pyridoxine and gestational diabetes recommend a reappraisal of the current RDA for pregnant women.[13]

Many pregnant women suffer from nausea. An Austrian doctor has found that these women, too, are often deficient in pyridoxine. By giving them 200 mg. supplements daily for a week, and 5 mg. per day afterwards, he found he could alleviate the nausea.[14]

Pyridoxine and Diabetes

If pyridoxine restores glucose tolerance in women with gestational diabetes, what would it do for diabetics? Diabetic adults and children do have lower blood levels of pyridoxine than people without diabetes. (This usually is inferred to indicate an increased demand for the vitamin.) In a group of 518 diabetic adults tested, twenty-five percent had blood levels of pyridoxine low enough to indicate a deficiency. Of 63 child diabetics tested, twenty-four percent had below-normal concentrations. This diabetic deficiency of pyridoxine is apparently too great to be overcome with diet alone.[15]

What is the significance of this deficiency? One study found that diabetics suffering from what is known as "diabetic neuropathy," which is a catchall term used to describe burning, pain, itching, cramping, restlessness, and loss of sensation and reflexes in the arms and legs, had even *lower* concentrations of pyridoxine in their blood than diabetics in general.[16]

If diabetic neuropathy appears very similar to the symptoms of a pyridoxine deficiency, you have noticed the same thing some Chicago doctors did. So for six weeks they gave supplements of 50 mg. of pyridoxine, three times a day, to a group of insulin-dependent diabetics who had neuropathy *and* evidence of pyridoxine deficiency. All their symptoms went away. Some doctors have also reported that pyridoxine reduces insulin requirements.[17]

Pyridoxine and Arthritis

There is practically no controversy over pyridoxine's ability to alleviate the depression sometimes brought on by oral contraceptives. Nor is there much disagreement surrounding its use in gestational diabetes or diabetic neuropathy. This is not to say the average doctor will know about these treatments, or that he will use them even if he does know. But there appears to be very little disagreement over whether the vitamin has the desired effect.

There is, however, a controversy regarding pyridoxine and arthritis. It appears that people with rheumatoid arthritis have impaired tryptophan metabolism and lower-than-normal blood levels of pyridoxine. These facts alone are enough to instigate a lot of speculation that arthritics might *need more* pyridoxine, and that if they get it, maybe their symptoms might lessen. The controversy intensifies here, because no one agrees whether the deficiency is due to some metabolic defect (which also might have something to do with the symptoms of the disease), or if it's merely caused by some of the *drugs* used to treat arthritis. One study did find that the deficiency was *not* related to drugs in rheumatoid arthritis, but that it *might be* in osteoarthritis (the drug used was Indomethacin).[18]

One study tried to answer *all* the questions by giving supplements of pyridoxine (50 to 150 mg.) to people with rheumatoid arthritis. Their pretreatment blood levels of pyridoxine were abnormally low. And although the blood levels came up beyond normal after supplementation, their arthritis symptoms did not respond.[19]

Dr. John M. Ellis, a Texas physician, has another point of view. Dr. Ellis probably knows more about what pyridoxine will and won't do than any other doctor or nutritionist. And Dr. Ellis says he's been successfully treating both what his *patients* call "rheumatism" and what *he* calls "rheumatism" with pyridoxine supplements. Dr. Ellis has seen hundreds of people with such symptoms as numbness, tingling, burning sensations in their extremities, fingers that "go to sleep," finger joints too stiff to form a proper fist, swelling of the fingers, reduced sensation in the fingers, leg cramps and "charley horses." Women have come in with "menopausal arthritis," with painful little red burrs or knots on the sides of their finger joints, in addition to some or all of the above symptoms. Sometimes the hand symptoms are joined by pain in the arms and shoulders.

These people invariably are given a supplement of pyridoxine (50 mg. per day). Within six weeks, according to Dr. Ellis, the symptoms are either gone or greatly improved. Swelling goes down, finger flexibility improves, cramps subside, numbness and tingling and pain in the joints of the fingers go away, and shoulder pain is reduced or eliminated.[20]

Dr. Ellis has also treated many people for something called "carpal tunnel syndrome," an inflammation of the nerves of the wrist, that leads to numbness, stiffness, pain, weakness, cramps, and nightly paralysis not only in the wrist but in the hand, fingers, arms, neck, and face. For many of his patients, this condition is bad enough to warrant surgery. Instead, Dr. Ellis treats them with large doses of pyridoxine (300 mg. per day), since his tests reveal they all suffer deficiencies. After two to four weeks, not only is the deficiency gone in most patients, but the symptoms are greatly relieved. Surgery becomes unnecessary, people can return to work, and most of them can go back to a normal life.[21]

Nutrition writers should always exercise caution when

dealing with information like this, lest people with serious, chronic diseases run into big disappointments when the nutritional therapy that "worked wonders" in print does little or nothing for them. Dr. Ellis's results are remarkable, and that is surely the least that any of the people he's helped would say. No doubt there are dozens, maybe hundreds, of doctors who not only have heard of Dr. Ellis's success with these symptoms of joint inflammation, but who are sharing it with some of their own patients.

Keep in mind, however, that Dr. Ellis may be splitting hairs when he calls their symptoms "rheumatism" instead of rheumatoid arthritis or arthritis. Keep in mind, also, that he tests his patients for biochemical evidence of pyridoxine deficiency, and that he generally finds it in those patients who are subsequently given pyridoxine supplements. A pyridoxine supplement is an easy, safe thing to take—many times safer than most arthritis drugs. But just as many people reading this might try adding more pyridoxine to their diets and find it helps them more than anything ever has before, many people might try pyridoxine and find nothing at all happens. (The same could be said, of course, for every beneficial effect mentioned in this book.)

Pyridoxine and Menstrual Symptoms

Pyridoxine may be of use to women who suffer depression and tension before their periods; however, the results of some experiments designed to test this have not been too encouraging. Still, pyridoxine does seem to do some good for some other premenstrual symptoms, such as swelling and acne, so it might be worth a try for tension and depression, too. Dr. Ellis's patients have had the same success with premenstrual swelling that they have had with "rheumatism," by using 100 mg. of pyridoxine per day.[22] And half that daily dose reduced the premenstrual acne flare-up of about seventy-five percent of a group of seventy-six teenagers.[23]

Apparently, pyridoxine can affect fertility in some women.

When a group of fourteen infertile women with premenstrual tension were given supplements of pyridoxine, ranging from 100 to 800 mg., for at least six months, twelve of them suddenly became fertile and conceived. High doses of pyridoxine are thought to suppress a hormone, prolactin, which not only stimulates lactation but also prevents fertility. This is the only clue we have as to why pyridoxine made these women fertile after they had been infertile for from eighteen months to seven years.[24]

Pyridoxine and Mental Illness

Orthomolecular psychiatrists sometimes use megadoses of pyridoxine in the treatment of schizophrenia. There are two reasons for this. One is that pyridoxine is known to be an important factor in the metabolism of niacin and tryptophan, both of which are also used in psychiatric therapy. The second reason is that some schizophrenics and other psychiatric patients excrete a substance which stains with the color *mauve* under a chromatogram analysis. This is called the "mauve factor." The mauve factor has been identified as a very toxic substance, *kryptopyrrole* (KP). KP *binds* pyridoxine, leading the doctors to believe that the presence of KP reveals an increased need for the vitamin.

Very high doses of pyridoxine, up to several grams a day, must be given to offset the mauve factor. But in many of these cases, the therapy is successful in alleviating the symptoms of schizophrenia. Some doctors give the pyridoxine along with high doses of niacin, vitamin C, and the minerals zinc and manganese.[25]

Pyridoxine and Children

Pyridoxine first became "famous" for its involvement in convulsions in newborn babies, as already described. But pyridoxine continues to be of use not only in the treatment of children and babies who suffer convulsions, but also in hyperactive and disturbed children.

Investigators found that children with the symptoms of hyperactivity—high activity, low frustration, impulsiveness, short attention span, and social unresponsiveness—had low levels of the neurotransmitter *serotonin* in their blood. They administered pyridoxine in hopes of raising the levels of this important brain chemical, since these low levels are thought to have some role in hyperactivity. The high doses of pyridoxine, which ranged from about 100 mg. to over 1000 mg. daily, did succeed in raising the serotonin levels. Unfortunately, the investigators did not record whether or not any behavioral changes were evident.[26] Their reluctance to do so suggests they wanted to avoid the controversy that would have arisen if pyridoxine's effects were reported to be beneficial. Hyperactivity is one of the principal battlefields of nutritional therapy and conventional drug therapy. Many doctors who successfully use nutritional therapy choose to avoid the battles and simply go on treating their patients with nutrition without "making waves."

Nonetheless, there is a published report of pyridoxine therapy alleviating hyperactive symptoms in a three-year-old girl. The child had a history of irritability, fussiness, and other minor ailments from the age of eleven months. At the age of three, the girl had a positive tuberculin skin test and was treated with *isoniazid*, an antituberculin drug. Shortly thereafter, her symptoms worsened. She couldn't sleep, she became irritable, hyperactive, and threw temper tantrums. Since isoniazid is known to interfere with pyridoxine metabolism, she was given a supplement of 100 mg. per day. Her symptoms *lessened*, but did not go away. Her supplement dose was raised to 400 mg. per day and the symptoms *disappeared*. After six months, both isoniazid and pyridoxine were discontinued. But the symptoms of hyperactivity returned. So she was again given 400 mg. of pyridoxine. Again, the symptoms disappeared. Whenever she was given a placebo instead of real pyridoxine, her symptoms returned in force within days.

Other drugs which apparently interfere with pyridoxine—sulfisoxazole or decongestants—have also brought the symptoms back. Her doctors have concluded that her hyperactivity was "unmasked" by the drugs, and that the increased need for pyridoxine *may* have always been present.[27]

Pyridoxine also has a beneficial effect for many children with *autism*. In a study of children whose autism appeared to be greatly improved when given pyridoxine, a placebo was substituted for the vitamin. During pyridoxine withdrawal, their behavior deteriorated significantly, as rated by parents and teachers. When the pyridoxine was resupplied, the improvement returned.[28]

A child doesn't have to be hyperactive or disturbed to benefit from pyridoxine. One pediatrician found that breath-holding spells (which are really harmless, but try to tell that to a parent whose child has just done it and passed out!) could be reduced or eliminated by daily supplements of 40 mg. a day for children up to two years old, and twice that amount for older children. The doctor reports that these children usually do have biochemical evidence of an increased need for pyridoxine.[29]

Pyridoxine and Heart Disease

Again, pyridoxine-deficient animals develop arteriosclerosis that is identical to the human disease. This is another one of those places where caution is well-advised before concluding the vitamin is either useless or omnipotent. No responsible physician or nutritionist would claim that pyridoxine deficiency is *the* cause of heart disease. There is simply too much evidence that our high fat and sugar diet and sedentary but competitive lifestyle are critically involved. Yet there is evidence that pyridoxine is also involved, and that supplying "adequate" amounts of the vitamin may be of *help* in preventing and treating the disease. But don't assume that someone can avoid heart disease simply by taking vitamin supplements. Such an assumption would be foolhardy.

Pyridoxine has a role in the formation of collagen. This role may apply to heart disease, because many doctors believe that the initial defect in heart disease is in the structure of the arteries, that the integrity of the vessels is damaged and that this lays the groundwork for later deposition of fat and minerals in the vessel. Some researchers believe that pyridoxine deficiency during pregnancy may cause this initial lesion, and that the generally poor nutritional quality of the average American diet perpetuates the deficiency and contributes to heart disease. There is enough evidence of the effects of maternal pyridoxine deficiency—and the prevalance of such deficiency is thought to be great enough—to require us to take this theory quite seriously.[30]

Unfortunately, the only published reports on this involve either animal experiments or biochemical data on humans. Is it possible that all the *other* factors which contribute to heart disease do so by interfering with pyridoxine metabolism, causing a greatly increased need for the vitamin? Not likely, although there may be a mixture of effects. Undoubtedly, pyridoxine is something that people should consider in the prevention and treatment of heart disease. But it shouldn't be the only thing.

Pyridoxine and Cancer

There is a lot of evidence that suggests that pyridoxine is involved in cancer. In women with advanced cancer of the breast and other sites, there is biochemical evidence of a deficiency or increased requirement for the vitamin. Dietary pyridoxine levels in these women are large enough to maintain adequate concentrations in the body, yet there is still a shortage. The implication is that pyridoxine is somehow "used up" in the body's defense against cancer, or that the disease merely interferes with pyridoxine metabolism. In persons with Hodgkin's Disease, biochemical signs of pyridoxine deficiency normalize when the disease goes into remission. The tantalizing question, and one that really has only begun to be tested, is whether supplementation with pyridoxine could have any effect on the course of the disease.[31]

In at least one study, relatively low-dosage supplementation (25 mg.) with pyridoxine slightly diminished *recurrence* of bladder tumors. When the people who didn't have recurrences during the first ten months of the study were eliminated from the calculations, the pyridoxine was found to have had a significantly stronger preventive effect than the conventional anticancer drug. Doctors theorized that the pyridoxine may have taken longer to take effect. This would be reasonable if the pyridoxine were actually strengthening the body's immune system.[32]

Pyridoxine and Toxic Chemicals

Pyridoxine protects the liver against acetaldehyde toxicity. If there is enough pyridoxine present, the protection is complete. The implication of this effect is that pyridoxine deficiency in the liver is a factor in liver diseases caused by certain toxins, such as alcohol.[33]

Pyridoxine also reverses the toxicity of *isoniazid*, a drug used in treating tuberculosis. About one in six people who take this drug develop the neuropathic symptoms of pyridoxine deficiency. A supplement of about 100 mg. is usually sufficient to alleviate the symptoms.[34] However, even people who take accidental or suicidal overdoses can be helped. In one report, a young man swallowed a whole bottle (fifteen to twenty tablets) of isoniazid and was brought to the hospital with severe convulsions. He was semicomatose when the doctors injected him with 100 mg. of pyridoxine. Within three hours he was alert, well-oriented, and stable.[35]

Hydrazine is another toxic chemical from which pyridoxine can protect us. Hydrazine is used in industry as a corrosion inhibitor and as a rocket propellant. People exposed to it in low levels over long periods of time develop pneumonia, liver damage, and inflammation of the kidneys. Exposure to large doses can cause seizures or coma. (If these symptoms sound similar to those of isoniazid toxicity, it's because isoniazid is chemically related to hydrazine.) Pyridoxine is an effective antidote to hydrazine poisoning in both animals and people. In one report, a man was exposed to hydrazine in an industrial explosion. He was in a coma for almost three days before doctors tried a large injected dose of pyridoxine. Within four hours, he was no longer comatose, and within twelve hours he was fully alert and functional.[36]

Pyridoxine has also been shown to reduce the side-effect syndrome of certain psychoactive drugs, called *tardive dyskinesia*. (See Choline chapter.) And, as we've seen, pyridoxine alleviates many of the side effects of oral contraceptives.

ARE WE GETTING ENOUGH PYRIDOXINE?

The RDA for pyridoxine ranges from .3 mg. for infants to 2.5 mg. for pregnant or lactating women. For adult males, the RDA is 2.2 mg.; for adult females, 2 mg. Considering the evidence in this chapter, there are probably more people who need *more* than that than there are who need less or who can get along with that much. Pyridoxine requirements vary not only with age, growth rate, and caloric intake, but with protein intake, too. The more protein you eat, the more pyridoxine you need to metabolize that protein.

Obviously, women taking oral contraceptives (and pregnant women) need to be extra careful they are getting enough pyridoxine, and that may not be possible without supplements. Pregnant women have been advised by many doctors to take vitamin-mineral supplements. A pyridoxine deficiency in pregnancy can have obvious symptoms to warn the woman, but it can also sneak up on her and go unnoticed until it is too late. One study measured the concentration of pyridoxine in the bodies of "healthy" pregnant women and found their vitamin status went lower and lower as the pregnancy progressed. The most rapid drop occurred during the period when the fetus was undergoing its most intense growth. This study also found that the higher the mother's pyridoxine levels before and during pregnancy, the higher the birthweight of their babies.[37]

Megadoses of pyridoxine are not required for pregnant women to maintain adequate body concentrations of pyridoxine. In one study, 10 mg. kept levels high throughout pregnancy. A supplement of this amount also resulted in high levels of the vitamin in the cord blood of the newborn babies.[38]

All women should probably take extra care with this vitamin, since they tend to have lower concentrations in their bodies than men. This is most likely an indication of increased utilization and need.

Perhaps men and women alike should watch their pyridoxine supply as they get older, since this same study revealed that pyridoxine blood and tissue levels decrease *with age,* too.[39] Other studies have confirmed the drop in pyridoxine status with age. About twenty-five percent of all people tested between the ages of eighteen and ninety had levels of pyridoxine low enough to indicate a deficiency.[40]

Among people who don't have any of the above predisposing conditions, pyridoxine deficiencies are still fairly common. One study of college students found that seventy-five percent of them did not get the RDA for pyridoxine in their diets.[41] Another study found that fourteen percent of a group of 341 schoolchildren had lower-than-normal blood levels of the vitamin.[42]

IS PYRIDOXINE TOXIC?

Pyridoxine is not considered especially toxic. Rats tolerate doses up to 1 gram per kilogram of body weight without effect. Above that amount, however, convulsions occur. A 4 to 6 gram dose can be lethal to rats. Extrapolating these doses to humans, it would take more than 50,000 milligrams to cause toxic symptoms in a person who weighed 100 pounds. All of the doses mentioned in this chapter, for all but the most serious diseases, were between 10 and 500 mg. For the severe diseases, doctors have used up to 5000 mg., which is well within safe limits.

Dr. Ellis reported no ill effects in any of the people he treated with pyridoxine, except in people with stomach ulcers. Nursing mothers should not take *high* supplements of pyridoxine, since doses of 600 mg. per day may suppress lactation. There are no other side effects from this high a dose.[44]

People being treated with tryptophan for depression should not take extra pyridoxine, unless they are deficient. Pyridoxine may *reverse* the beneficial effects tryptophan has on depression by stimulating the conversion of tryptophan to niacin. Pyridoxine may also interfere with the drug *levodopa* used in Parkinsonism.[45]

SOURCES OF PYRIDOXINE

The richest natural sources of pyridoxine include liver and other organ meats, whole-grain cereals, wheat germ, soybeans, yeast, peanuts, corn, and blackstrap molasses. Some fruits and vegetables are also good sources, including cabbage, bananas, potatoes, avocadoes, peas, and green peppers. Since pyridoxine is water-soluble and sensitive to light, many canning and processing procedures destroy substantial amounts of it. Vegetable sources of the vitamin should be eaten raw for maximum benefit.

There is some evidence that wheat bran may "soak up" some pyridoxine and cause it to be excreted. If you eat a lot of wheat bran, you should make sure you're getting enough pyridoxine, preferably at other meals than those at which you eat bran.

Although some of the best sources of pyridoxine are meats, a study of pyridoxine levels in vegans (people who eat no animal products at all) and meat-eaters found no significant differences between the two groups.[43]

Pyridoxine is available in supplements in a wide range of doses, from 5 mg. to over 500 mg.

6

Folate

We take for granted that our wounds will heal, that our mental health will survive the daily stresses of modern living, and that we'll have enough energy to get us through the day. Yet when these systems start to falter, we often don't acknowledge the fact that something's wrong. We grow accustomed to wounds that seem to take forever to heal. We blame our irritability and nervousness on other people. We admit we're "just getting older" when the day starts to seem too long.

But we ignore the fact that what's really happening is we're sliding away from optimum health.

Folate (also known as folacin and folic acid) plays an important role in many of the systems which are vital to maintaining our position on the continuum.

WHAT FOLATE DOES

Though folate's exact role in metabolism is not yet fully

known, we know it's necessary for the synthesis of essential nucleic acids, DNA and RNA. These proteins are required for cell reproduction and division, so it doesn't take much imagination to realize how devastating a deficiency of this vitamin could be. The "hardest hit" target organs are those that depend on rapid proliferation of new cells: bone marrow, hair, fingernails, immune system, certain mucous membranes, and red blood cells.

Take a look at some of these areas right now. Are you satisfied with the health of your hair and fingernails? Let's put it this way: can you remember a time when they were in better shape?

Now, there are certainly many reasons why your hair or fingernails might not be in as good a condition as you might like them to be. But one of those possible reasons is the state of your folate supply. Of course, it's not quite so easy to examine the health of your bone marrow, red blood cells, mucous membranes, or immune system. But if your hair and nails aren't what you know they can be, it's possible that a folate defect in your nutrition is impairing these important organ systems.

WHAT HAPPENS WHEN
FOLATE DEMAND EXCEEDS SUPPLY

The dominant physiological effect of a folate deficiency appears to be its effect on the production of new red blood cells. When the required proteins are not supplied, the new cells do not properly mature and are stuck in the *megaloblast* stage. Megaloblastic red blood cells are too big to adequately perform the function of red blood cells, which is to deliver oxygen to the cells. Anemia results, along with a decrease in the number of blood platelets and leukocytes (white blood cells) in the blood.

Folate deficiency also has devastating effects upon the nervous system. Concentrations of folate are normally much higher in the spinal fluid than in the blood.[1] Such a concentration in a particular organ usually means the nutrient is somehow very important to the structure and function of that organ. In this case, the relation holds true, because the effects of a folate deficiency can appear "indistinguishable from degeneration of the spinal cord."[2]

This is a controversial area, because the standard view of folate deficiency is that anemia occurs *without* degeneration of the nervous system, despite the mountain of evidence that folate deficiency *is* involved in damage to the nervous system. Many nutritionists and doctors maintain that only a deficiency of cobalamin (B_{12}) produces an anemia which damages the nervous system, and that supplying folate when there is a cobalamin deficiency (pernicious anemia) can "mask" the damage to the nervous system while seeming to cure the anemia. Apparently, the same may also occur if only cobalamin is supplied during a folate deficiency.

A folate deficiency also affects the immune system. Several studies have demonstrated that a folate deficiency impairs *cellular immunity*, which is the most basic part of the immune system. In animals maintained on a folate-free diet, lymphocyte (white blood cell) activity is markedly reduced.[3] The same appears to occur in people. Studies of people with megaloblastic anemia have revealed that lymphocyte activity is impaired and that folate supplementation quickly restores the cellular immune system to normal function. The cellular immune system is responsible for our resistance to viral, fungal, parasitic, and certain bacterial infections.[4]

Symptoms

The classic symptoms of a folate deficiency anemia are weakness, inflamed and sore tongue, numbness or tingling in the hands and feet, indigestion, diarrhea, depression, irritability, pallor, drowsiness, and slow, weakened pulse. These are also the symptoms of pernicious anemia, which is due to a deficiency of cobalamin (B_{12})

As with most of the other vitamins and minerals, these

"classic" symptoms are revealed experimentally by means of severe deprivation. Remember that the continuum contains a wide range of illness and health. There is no cut-off point where a difference between supply and demand suddenly becomes severe enough to be called a deficiency and cause these symptoms. As soon as supply does not meet demand, there is going to be a biochemical effect. The adverse effect on optimum health may be slight, but it will occur nevertheless. Wounds may not heal as fast as they should. Hair might fall out in greater than normal volume. Infections might take hold more frequently than before. Then, some of the "classic" symptoms may show up.

Folate and Mental Illness

Folate deficiency can produce clinically observable and measurable signs of *polyneuropathy*, which means disease or inflammation of the nerves. The symptoms are weakness in the extremities, reduction or loss of reflexes, loss of feeling in the extremities, difficulty in walking or using the arms, and cramps. Such symptoms are signs that the nervous system, especially the spinal cord, is being impaired or damaged. Folate supplementation in relatively high doses can alleviate these symptoms.[5]

But can folate deficiency affect the *brain*? Can your folate supply make a difference in your everyday mental functioning?

Apparently it can. One study of 269 psychiatric patients in a hospital found that folate deficiency was more frequent than it was among people admitted to the hospital for other reasons. The range of mental symptoms in these patients included forgetfulness, apathy, irritability, insomnia, delirium, depression, psychosis, dementia, and mental retardation. The investigators who carried out this study felt that these deficiencies were not the result of bad diet *alone*, but that some people have increased requirements for folate because of internal enzymatic defects.[6] Other investigators have found that impairment of brain function is more common among persons with folate deficiency than among those with no deficiency.[7]

One courageous physician placed *himself* on a folate-deficient diet and noted the psychological changes as the deficiency took hold. After four to five months of the deficiency, sleeplessness, forgetfulness, and irritability appeared and became gradually worse. When he restored folate to his diet, his symptoms disappeared within forty-eight hours.[8]

If sleeplessness, forgetfulness, and irritability are chronic problems for you, the simplest way to tell if a folate deficiency is the cause is to increase the amount of folate in your diet.

One researcher found that folate deficiency resulting from either malabsorption, deficient diet, or metabolic defect could result in atrophy of the brain and mental disorders. The symptoms were much the same as in other reports of folate deficiency: depression, muscular weakness, intellectual fatigue, restless legs syndrome, depressed reflexes and loss of feeling in the extremities. The people ranged in age from twenty-six to seventy-six. When folate supplements were administered, their intellectual functioning strikingly improved.[9]

The same investigator treated six women, age thirty-one to seventy, who had these same symptoms. One of the women, age forty-four, had a three-year history of unrelenting fatigue, depression, and numbness in the legs. Daily housework and care of her two children had grown impossible for her. She had suffered headaches every evening for the past four years. Dizziness and blurred vision plagued her during the day. Understandably, she had a lot of anxiety. She also had biochemical evidence of a folate deficiency. She was given 5 to 10 mg. of folate orally per day, plus an injection of folate once a week. Her depression disappeared and her headaches and other symptoms decreased remarkably. She was able to return to a normal life. The same kind of success stories could be told for the other women treated with folate.[10]

Folate has also helped schizophrenia patients recover. In a British study, patients with folate deficiencies and mental disorders—schizophrenia, depression, and psychosis—were divided into two groups. One group was given folate supplements and the other was not. The group that got the supplements was discharged from the hospital substantially sooner than those not given them. The group not given folate spent from twenty to fifty percent longer in the mental hospital.[11] There have been other reports of individual schizophrenics being helped by folate.[12]

Occasionally, the neurological impairment caused by a folate deficiency will be labeled "senility." A British study found that ten elderly patients in a hospital suffering from a confused mental condition were all deficient in folate.[13] Another study found that thirty-five percent of a group of elderly patients with confusion, disorientation, depression, hallucinations, delusions, alcohol intoxication or withdrawal symptoms, and bodily preoccupation had folate deficiencies. This study revealed the value of a good diet in preventing these problems in old age, for another group of elderly people *without* mental symptoms was tested and surveyed. All had good dietary habits and none had folate deficiencies.[14]

Folate and Low Blood Sugar

Folate apparently helps maintain normal blood sugar levels. Folate-supplemented rats had higher blood sugar levels after a forty-eight-hour fast than rats which did not fast but received no folate.[15] Apparently this effect has therapeutic value for some people who suffer from chronic low blood sugar. A twenty-eight-year-old woman and her nineteen-month-old daughter were treated for hypoglycemia with folate supplements (5 mg., three times per day; this much folate should never be given a child except under a physician's observation). Before treatment, the mother was easily fatigued, depressed, or angered. She was unable to do housework without stopping to rest, and she would just sit down and cry frequently, with no apparent reason. Alternating sweats and chills and dizziness occurred from two to five hours after meals. During the glucose tolerance test, she displayed all of these symptoms, as many classic cases of hypoglycemia do. Her baby daughter's symptoms were occasional confusion and disorientation. She would wake up crying frequently in the middle of the night.

Folate treatment greatly improved the condition of both mother and daughter. They were better able to maintain normal blood levels of glucose, and their symptoms decreased or disappeared. Although folate deficiency is not usually considered a cause of hypoglycemia, these people apparently had a defect in an enzyme system that required folate. The doctors who treated them suggested that such an enzymatic defect might be a cause of hypoglycemia in people who are not helped by the standard methods of treatment.[16]

Folate and Heart Disease

Cardiologist Kurt Oster, M.D., has formulated one of the most intriguing theories of heart disease: Dr. Oster says atherosclerosis is caused by an enzyme, *xanthine oxidase*, which enters the body through the digestive tract and attacks the linings of the arteries. Cholesterol, and ultimately, calcium, are deposited in the lesions, and atherosclerosis results.

Where does the villainous enzyme come from? *Cow's milk.* Dr. Oster has done extensive epidemiological studies and has shown that heart disease is more common in countries that drink a lot of homogenized milk. Homogenization, he believes, makes the enzyme more biologically available, and thus more lethal. The answer to heart disease, he says, is to drink less homogenized milk and to treat people with heart disease by *neutralizing* the xanthine oxidase. Although other chemicals are available that will neutralize xanthine oxidase, Dr. Oster chose folate because of its nontoxicity. He gives his heart patients 40 to 80 mg. per day, and has done so for almost ten years. The ones who keep up with the treatment and continue to take the folate have less need for nitroglycerin to control their angina and have fewer heart attacks than those who don't take folate, according to Dr. Oster.

Dr. Oster appears to know what he's talking about. He

takes folate himself for his own heart condition. He is roundly attacked by the "heart disease establishment," and he just as roundly attacks back. His treatment may very well have benefit. But, again, remember that a single vitamin or mineral is not the answer to heart disease. There is too much good evidence, such as Dr. Oster's, that vitamins and minerals *are* important. But if you believe *every* one is *the* answer, you will be left quite confused with all these single "answers" to a very vexing problem.

Besides, Dr. Oster's treatment is impractical at this time, since he has a special license from the FDA to allow him to prescribe folate in such large doses. You probably could not get such high doses unless you went to Canada, or talked your cardiologist into getting another special license from the FDA.[17]

Folate and Psoriasis

An unexpected bonus from Dr. Oster's work has been that psoriasis may respond to folate supplements. Seven of his patients with psoriasis were given 80 mg. of folate per day in four equally divided doses. Within three to six months, their skin was "almost normal." Dr. Oster's rationale behind using folate was that it restores *plasmologen*, a cellular substance the disease attacks.[18] Dr. Oster may be on the right track, because other researchers have found folate levels low in people with psoriasis.[19] In some studies, the greater the extent of the lesion, the greater the correlation with folate levels.[20]

Folate and Gingivitis

Folate evidently benefits the health of the gums. In one study, fifteen people ranging in age from nineteen to fifty-eight were given 2 mg. supplements of folate per day. Another group of fifteen was given a placebo. All subjects were rated for gingival health at the beginning and after thirty days. The people who had received folate had a fifty percent decrease in gingival exudate flow, a reliable indicator of gum inflammation. No change was seen in the people who received no folate. None of the people had biochemical evidence of a folate deficiency at the start of the study, so the doctors concluded that the supplementary folate was correcting a local deficiency at the "end organ" site—the gums.[21]

These same researchers found that a folate solution *rinse*, five minutes twice a day, could also substantially reduce both inflammation and bleeding in the gums.[22] They also found that oral contraceptives could cause these "end organ" deficiencies in women's gums, and that folate supplementation could overcome that deficiency and reduce inflammation.[23]

Folate and Pregnancy

Because it is required for the manufacture of new tissue, folate is vitally important to not only the health of the pregnant woman but also to the proper development of the fetus. As we shall see, a folate deficiency during pregnancy can have devastating effects.

One of the relatively minor effects, however, is something called "restless legs" syndrome. The symptoms—insomnia, leg numbness and cramps which are relieved by movement and massage of the calves—generally come during the night. One study found restless legs syndrome was directly associated with low dietary and blood levels of folate. Out of a group of twenty-one pregnant women, nine had restless leg syndrome. Only one of these women had received a folate supplement. Of the other twelve, who didn't have restless leg syndrome, ten had taken folate supplements.[24]

A folate deficiency can seriously affect the developing fetus. In one study of over 700 women with spontaneous abortions, over a third of the women who suffered abortions more than once had low blood levels of folate. This percentage is seven times what you would expect it to be if folate had nothing to do with their abortions. Another study of over 800 women found that fetal malformations in the 135 women with low folate levels were four times more frequent than in the 670 women with normal values. Central nervous system defects have been found to be equally more frequent in infants born to mothers with folate deficiency.[25] And infants born with immature red blood cells, a result of maternal folate deficiency, were found to have lower birthweight and retarded growth.[26] Occasionally, such a child will display symptoms of retarded motor development. Such a "floppy" infant was reported unable to sit, stand, or roll over at the age of seven months. This child was fortunate in that her doctors gave her supplements of folate, and by the time she was a year old, her motor development had practically caught up and her mental development was normal.[27]

Folate deficiency during pregnancy can have neurological effects on the mother as well. "Baby blues," or what doctors call "post-partum psychosis," can be a result of folate deficiency. One woman went through hell before her doctors finally discovered she was suffering from a folate deficiency. After her baby was born, she became increasingly withdrawn, irritable, and depressed. She often became confused, paranoid, panicky, and agitated. She hallucinated monsters that were after her and her baby. She was hospitalized and underwent eight courses of electroshock therapy. She was transferred to a state hospital and treated with tranquilizers and other psychiatric drugs; she got worse instead of better. She was released from the hospital because her family could no longer bear her isolation in a "seclusion room" at the hospital. Her symptoms grew worse and more frequent. She was hospitalized after each one of three separate suicide attempts. After the third attempt, numerous biochemical tests were performed and she was found not only to have macrocytic anemia but *no detectable* folate in her blood. So finally, almost two years after her ordeal began, she was given high doses of folate (5 mg. twice a day, injected into the muscles), and within a *week* her mental status began to improve! *By the tenth day* she was completely well. She was released from the hospital with a prescription for 1 mg. of folate a day, and at the time of the report two and

a half years later, she had no recurrence of mental disturbances. As a matter of fact, she was reported to be doing very
well in school.[28]

Such a story speaks for itself regarding the relationship of
folate to mental health and a healthy pregnancy. It's quite
evident that pregnancy raises a woman's requirement for
folate. And the reports of just *how many* women have been
found deficient are scary. In a study of low-income pregnant
women in New York City, sixteen percent were found with
folate deficiencies low enough to suggest "tissue depletion,"
and a further fourteen percent had marginal levels.[29] A study
of a small group of women who were from higher economic
levels, however, found over *half* with evidence of at least a
mild deficiency.[30]

These reports of what a folate deficiency can do to a mother
and her baby, coupled with the apparently widespread incidence of folate deficiencies, do not make for very encouraging
comment upon the state of our nutrition *or* the quality of
prenatal care. Especially when you consider that it generally
takes a scant *half milligram*, or .5 mg., of folate to prevent
those deficiencies. In a British study, half a milligram did just
as well as 5 milligrams in alleviating and preventing folate
deficiency in a small group of women tested. This doesn't
mean all women need that little; some may need much more.
But it does demonstrate how easy it would be to eliminate a
lot of suffering.[31]

REQUIREMENTS FOR FOLATE

The RDA for folate ranges from .05 mg. for infants up to .8
mg. for pregnant women. For adults, the RDA is .4 mg.
Reference books admit that the human requirement has not
yet been adequately determined. But the same could be said
for just about any vitamin, considering the wide variations in
individual needs. It seems much more folate is generally
needed to overcome individual deficiencies. And it would
appear that a great many people need to overcome deficiencies.

Oral contraceptives can cause folate deficiencies, and the deficiencies can linger for many months after contraceptives are no longer taken.[32]

In Canada, up to thirteen percent of the population is estimated to be at high risk for folate deficiency, and about thirty-two to fifty-nine percent at moderate risk.[33]

In a study of 110 teenage girls and 87 pregnant women, the mean dietary folate intake was found to be less than one-third of the RDA.[34] In a study of 341 schoolchildren, 42 had deficient blood levels of folate.[35] One group that was found to have sufficient folate stores was breastfed infants.[36]

Folate deficiencies are apparently quite common in hospital patients. (This is not extraordinary, since the hospital is a breeding ground for malnutrition.) In forty-six long-term elderly patients studied in one hospital, folate intake was found to be inadequate in most.[37] Another study documented severe deterioration of folate status of 129 consecutive hospital patients from the day of admission.[38] And many cases of severe folate deficiency develop in hospital patients receiving intravenous nutrition, which is often in an alcohol solution unsupplemented with vitamins. Some have almost led to the death of the victims.[39]

Many commonly used drugs interfere with folate metabolism and could cause deficiencies. Oral contraceptives increase the removal of folate from the blood plasma; methotrexate, a drug used for immunosuppression in cancer and psoriasis, is a folate antagonist. Other drugs which can interfere with folate are aminopterin, the antimalarial drug pyrimethamine, pentamidine, trimethoprim, phenytoin, primidone, phenobarbitone, isoniazid and cycloserine combination therapy, alcohol, diphenylhydantoin, barbiturates, estrogens, anticonvulsants, and phenothiazines.[40]

Folate depletion occurs rapidly after injury or trauma.[41] Absorption of folate is impaired by a systemic bacterial infection.[42] And people with sickle cell anemia frequently have a folate deficiency.[43] Folate absorption from the intestine is impaired in a zinc deficiency.[44] Vitamin C is necessary for the conversion of folate to its biologically active form, so folate deficiency can occur as a result of a vitamin C deficiency.[45]

IS FOLATE TOXIC?

Folate is relatively nontoxic. Animals must be given the human equivalent of many thousands of milligrams before any signs of toxicity occur. Extra high doses in humans can sometimes cause gastrointestinal upset, irritability, altered sleep pattern, vivid dreaming, nervousness, and hyperactivity. These symptoms show up at doses that would be available only from a special prescription.[46]

The administration of cobalamin along with folate may prevent the above symptoms and should be routine.

Other precautions: folate should be given only with great caution to epileptic people, since the vitamin can interfere with epileptic drugs. And since folate stimulates RNA and DNA, doctors advise cancer patients not to take large doses.[47]

SOURCES OF FOLATE

Rich natural sources of folate include organ meats, dark green leafy vegetables, asparagus, lima beans, yeast, whole grains, wheat germ, lentils, and orange juice. From fifty to ninety-five percent of folate can be destroyed by cooking, canning, processing, or storage, since the vitamin is sensitive to sunlight, heat, and acids.

In the United States, folate supplements are available in doses only up to .8 mg. The dose in a single tablet is regulated, because folate is believed to mask the anemia symptoms of pernicious anemia (a cobalamin deficiency) while allowing the neurological deterioration of the disease to continue. A more rational solution would be merely to alert physicians and nutritionists to the need to administer *both* vitamins in suspicious cases of anemia, rather than denying a much larger segment of the population access to a vitamin many surely need in larger doses. In Canada and other foreign countries, folate is available in higher doses.

7

Cobalamin (B$_{12}$)

Whenever an omnivore and a vegetarian argue the relative merits of eating no animal products, the omnivore is likely to pull out cobalamin as a vampire hunter might brandish garlic or a crucifix. Because cobalamin's primary natural sources are animal products, a strict vegetarian (vegan) is theoretically unable to get enough cobalamin without resorting to supplements. Hence, vegetarianism is neither as "safe" nor as "natural" as vegetarians think it is.

This, of course, obscures the fact that there's evidence we omnivores are no better off than the vegetarians and that getting more cobalamin in our diets might move us all closer to optimum health.

WHAT COBALAMIN DOES

Also known as cyanocobalamin and B$_{12}$, cobalamin is the largest molecule of all the vitamins. It is unique in that it is the only vitamin to contain a metal, *cobalt*. Because of its complexity, cobalamin was not synthesized until 1972.

Like folate, cobalamin is an essential participant in nucleic acid synthesis. Cobalamin is also essential to the metabolism of folate, and is essential to the structure and function of the nervous system.

Cobalamin absorption from the gastrointestinal tract is almost nonexistent unless another substance, called the *intrinsic factor*, is also present. Intrinsic factor is a glycoprotein which is secreted by a normal, healthy stomach. If the intrinsic factor is not present, very large doses of cobalamin (more than .025 mg.) will be only partially absorbed. Other proteins are necessary for transport of the vitamin in the blood and uptake by the cells. These proteins are called *transcobalamines*.

The cause of cobalamin deficiency (pernicious anemia) is usually the lack of intrinsic factor, not dietary lack of the vitamin. People with pernicious anemia have been found to excrete large amounts of the vitamin when it is given them, indicating that it is not being absorbed.

Animals can synthesize cobalamin (or rather, the bacteria in their gastrointestinal tract can synthesize it), utilizing dietary cobalt. Humans cannot do this, however, and must rely on a dietary source. The only cobalt the human body uses is that which enters via cobalamin.

WHAT HAPPENS WHEN COBALAMIN DEMAND EXCEEDS SUPPLY

Again, like folic acid, a deficiency of cobalamin impairs the formation of red blood cells. The red blood cells are halted at the immature megaloblast (large cell) stage. The nervous system is also affected, with deterioration of structure and function. Untreated, pernicious anemia is ultimately fatal. Until the cure was discovered in 1926, the disease killed more than 6000 Americans every year.

Pernicious anemia *can* result from a dietary lack of cobalamin, but evidence suggests it's more often from some defect in the person's digestion which results in either a deficit of intrinsic factor or in the production of substances which destroy or render the intrinsic factor useless. Specific antibodies to the intrinsic factor have been found in the gastric juice, saliva, and blood of people with pernicious anemia. The disease rapidly responds to injections of cobalamin or administration of the vitamin with the intrinsic factor. Administering folate in cases of pernicious anemia will alleviate the signs of anemia in the blood, but will not necessarily halt the neurological deterioration. But since folate deficiency also produces similar and equally damaging anemia and nervous system damage, it's important that a physician or a nutritionist either administer both or be accurate in determining which vitamin is needed.

A deficiency of cobalamin also impairs the function of the small intestine, thus reducing the absorption of essential nutrients.[1] Blood platelet function is also impaired, resulting in extended bleeding time before clotting takes place. When the deficiency is corrected, clotting can sometimes occur *too* frequently and result in thrombosis.[2] Cobalamin deficiency can also mask a simultaneous iron deficiency by keeping blood levels of iron deceptively high. When the cobalamin deficiency is corrected, the iron deficiency becomes apparent in the blood.[3]

Cobalamin deficiency can sometimes cause visual difficulty and reduced color perception. Tobacco smoking can affect cobalamin levels, since many people with optic neuropathy associated with smoking also have cobalamin deficiencies. Tobacco smoking may lower absorption of the vitamin.[4]

In animal experiments, it has been shown that a cobalamin deficiency lowers brain levels of the neurotransmitter norepinephrine. This may account for some of the neurological effects of a deficiency.[5] Some researchers believe that the neurological effects of cobalamin deficiency are due to a disturbance of *folate* metabolism. It's known that a cobalamin deficiency *seriously* interferes with folate utilization, and it has been shown in recent research that folate deficiency results in neurological damage identical to that in cobalamin deficiency. This might explain why folate doesn't alleviate the neurological impairment of pernicious anemia: without adequate cobalamin, folate cannot be utilized.[6]

Symptoms of a Cobalamin Deficiency

The symptoms of pernicious anemia include weakness, sore and inflamed tongue, numbness and tingling in the extremities, pallor, weak pulse, stiffness, drowsiness, irritability, depression, and diarrhea.

Pernicious anemia, however, does not always result from a deficiency of cobalamin, not even severe deficiencies. A marginal deficiency could be expected to produce lesser versions of the above symptoms. And any person who suffers such symptoms on a day-to-day basis should first of all suspect some form of nutritional deficit.

However, other symptoms, ranging from mental problems to increased susceptibility to infections, can result. Certain organs or organ systems may be more susceptible to shortfalls in the supply of nutrients, from person to person. Two people with the same diet may suffer totally different symptoms. And a third person might appear perfectly healthy.

Cobalamin and Mental Health

Cobalamin appears to play a role in mental health independent of the dementia associated with pernicious anemia. Some people apparently have nervous systems which need more cobalamin to stay healthy. A severe deficiency can land them in the mental hospital, while a marginal deficiency may be just enough to make them very hard to get along with.

A Norwegian study found that more than fifteen percent of the patients admitted to a mental hospital over the course of a year had blood levels of cobalamin low enough to be considered deficient.[7] There are numerous reports of various mental disturbances successfully treated with cobalamin.

One of the most interesting is that of an eleven-year-old girl who was "accidentally" cured of psychosis. Her parents took her to the doctor after she started hearing voices calling her name. She was irritable, paranoid, moody, and uncooperative. Because she refused to take any medications, the doctor gave her cobalamin tablets to take twice a day. The idea was to substitute a psychiatric drug after the child grew accustomed to taking a pill twice a day. When she was brought back to the doctor a month later, it was no longer necessary to give her the drug. The vitamin had cured her psychosis. At the time of the report one year after the first treatment, the girl was still maintaining good mental health while taking 75 to 125 micrograms of cobalamin twice a day. When she didn't take the vitamin for a few days, her symptoms returned. The doctor reports that subsequent patients have been helped by cobalamin, too.[8]

Another report concerns a man who tried to commit suicide. He had been depressed, impotent, lacking libido, and forgetful. After a battery of tests—some of which the doctors admitted indicated a cobalamin deficiency—the young man was given tranquilizers. They didn't work. Ten courses of electroshock therapy didn't do the trick, either. The young man remained apathetic and confused, and added the new symptom of paranoia. (Considering what the doctors were doing to him, the paranoia seems justified!) After five months of trying drugs and other treatments, the young man was finally given cobalamin. His doctors called his response "dramatic." Eight days later he was discharged, with a complete disappearance of symptoms. He has remained well with monthly cobalamin injections.[9]

These reports were not isolated reports. Many other researchers and physicians have documented the relationship between mental illness and cobalamin deficiency. And various studies have surveyed people with pernicious anemia and found anywhere from three to sixty-four percent of them with mental disorders.[10]

Finally, one interesting study found that two injections of

cobalamin per week increased several people's self-ratings of their sense of well-being. The subjects were selected because they constantly complained of tiredness, but were not found to be deficient in the vitamin. Placebo injections did not have the same effect.[11]

Cobalamin and the Immune Response

A cobalamin deficiency impairs the activity of the immune system, primarily by inhibiting the leukocytes (the white and clear blood cells). *Phagocytosis*, the devouring of invading organisms by the leukocytes, was reduced to slightly more than one-third of normal. Bacterial killing was decreased, too. Supplementation with the vitamin reversed these effects.[12]

In another report, a young man's *herpes simplex* lesions on his penis and in his mouth would not heal with a treatment of vitamin C. However, the lesions healed when he was given cobalamin (.5 mg.).[13]

Cobalamin and Pregnancy

Fertility researchers have discovered that infertility can result from cobalamin deficiency without necessarily exhibiting the signs and symptoms of pernicious anemia.[14]

Doctors have found that an inborn defect in cobalamin metabolism, which usually results in a severely ill baby, can be treated by administering cobalamin in large doses to a pregnant woman known to be carrying a child with the defect. A woman who had lost her first baby to this defect was treated with the vitamin before giving birth to her second child. The child was born in "excellent condition," and subsequently placed on a maintenance dose of cobalamin.[15]

Higher than "adequate" levels of cobalamin may benefit healthy fetuses, too. In animal experiments, one group of pregnant animals was placed on a diet containing the "standard" recommended amount of cobalamin. A second group was given the standard diet, but with higher amounts of cobalamin. After giving birth, all were placed on the standard diet. The offspring of the females who had received extra cobalamin were heavier at birth, grew faster, had more resistance to infection, and had better survival rates than the animals whose mothers had received "standard" amounts.[16]

REQUIREMENTS FOR COBALAMIN

The RDA for cobalamin ranges from .3 micrograms (.0003 mg.) for infants to 4 micrograms (.004 mg.) for pregnant women. For adults, the RDA is .3 micrograms. These ranges are much lower than the doses used therapeutically. If a deficiency is based on dietary lack, improving the diet or supplementation will correct it. However, many deficiencies appear to be from a metabolic defect or a lack of intrinsic factor. In such cases, the intrinsic factor must be taken with any supplement, or the vitamin must be injected in order to bypass faulty absorption. People who have such a metabolic defect usually require one or the other of these treatments for life.[17]

There *are*, however, factors other than metabolic defects which can result in a cobalamin deficiency.

Some doctors and nutritionists love to point the finger at vegetarians and vegans as the people most likely to suffer a dietary cobalamin deficiency. The reason for this is that the primary sources of cobalamin are animal products. Now, there *are* sporadic reports of vegetarians and vegans with cobalamin deficiencies. One such report involved the baby of a vegetarian couple. The infant did have an obvious dietary lack of cobalamin and was suffering the consequences (pallor, floppiness) when her parents brought her to the emergency room. And cobalamin supplements made her well immediately. In this case, the parents weren't really very knowledgeable about nutrition: when a naturopath they consulted previously recommended they give the baby salt tablets and herbal tea, they did it. Naturally, the baby didn't improve. Then they brought her to the hospital emergency room.[18]

Vegetarians and vegans are generally much better educated in what nutrients they need and where to get them than most omnivores. Whatever the reason, the fact is that most vegetarians—whether smarter or luckier—don't display any of the symptoms of cobalamin deficiency. This may be because their bodies reach some kind of balance between need and supply in which their needs diminish, or because they simply utilize what they do get more efficiently.[19]

A person is much more likely to develop a cobalamin deficiency on a *hospital* diet than on a vegetarian diet. At least one study has reported cobalamin intake to be "borderline" in hospital diets.[20] Many drugs can cause a deficiency, too, including methotrexate, cholestyramine, neomycin, colchicine, sodium aminosalicylate, slow-release potassium chloride, metformin, phenformin, sodium nitroprusside, oral contraceptives and other estrogens, and alcohol.[21]

Elderly people are possible candidates for cobalamin deficiency, since our intrinsic factor secretion diminishes with age.[22] At least one study has found low blood levels of the vitamin among the elderly. Out of 273 geriatric hospital patients, one-third had deficient blood concentrations of cobalamin. Only 12 were due to malabsorption or metabolic defect. The rest (78) were caused by a dietary deficiency of folate or cobalamin.[23]

Finally, a few years ago a report was published and widely publicized which stated that high levels of vitamin C in the blood or diet could destroy cobalamin. The researcher who reported this discovered, however, that the cobalamin had been destroyed not by the vitamin C itself but by the heat of the blender used to mix the two. He promptly published a retraction, which was somewhat less widely publicized. Subsequent investigations by other researchers have confirmed that vitamin C in no way interferes with cobalamin.[24]

IS COBALAMIN TOXIC?

Cobalamin is not toxic. Injections of the vitamin as high as

5,000 to 10,000 times the usual therapeutic dose have been administered for three months without toxic effect.

SOURCES OF COBALAMIN

Organ meats are the best sources of cobalamin; muscle meats and fish supply it in moderate amounts, milk in somewhat smaller amounts. There *are* some vegetable sources: sea vegetables (seaweed such as wakame and kombu) and fermented soybeans (tempeh). Nutritional yeast can be grown on a cobalamin-fortified base, and the resultant yeast will provide cobalamin. Some yeasts are fortified with synthetic cobalamin, too.

Cobalamin is sensitive to light, acids, and alkalies. It is normally not destroyed in cooking; however, overheating may destroy it.

Cobalamin is available in supplements ranging from a few micrograms up to a milligram (1000 micrograms).

8

Biotin

One of the most fascinating stories of a vitamin deficiency concerns a man who actually became *addicted* to raw eggs and wine. That's right: *raw eggs and wine!* He was so enamored of these two items that he left his family and moved to a chicken farm where he'd always have plenty of raw eggs. He ate raw eggs and wine for breakfast, lunch, and dinner. When he wanted some variety, he skipped a meal. When he *really* wanted a change, he ate some canned food.

Finally, he ended up in a hospital—although it was for removal of a tumor, not for the symptoms of a vitamin deficiency. When his doctors asked him about his severely reddened skin and his scaly dermatitis, he said his skin had always looked that way, although it *had* gotten somewhat worse over the past few years. As bad as hospital food can be, it's better than raw eggs and wine. The man's deficiency was corrected fairly quickly, with the assistance of vitamin supplements.

The man is reported to have remarked to his doctors that

his skin hadn't looked so good since he had been a teenager, about a half century before.[1]

This man was suffering what has come to be called "egg white injury." A substance in raw egg white, *avidin*, binds with the B vitamin biotin and renders it unavailable to the body. The man's love of raw eggs did him in by causing a severe biotin deficiency. Many nutritionists claim that egg white injury is the *only* way a biotin deficiency can occur; apparently this is not so. Other factors can cause our biotin supply to fall short of the demand, and cause us to slip backwards on the continuum.

WHAT BIOTIN DOES

Biotin's name comes from the Greek word for life, *bios*. Although biotin has been known to be essential for half a century, research has not yet fully revealed all of its roles. We know it is essential for the synthesis of protein and fatty acids, and to the metabolism of carbohydrates. In additon, biotin is an essential coenzyme in many enzyme reactions. We know that the thyroid and adrenal glands, the reproductive tract, the nervous system, and the skin depend on an adequate supply of the vitamin.

WHAT HAPPENS WHEN DEMAND EXCEEDS SUPPLY

A deficiency of biotin in animals results in severe dermatitis, hair loss, neuromuscular disorders, deterioration of heart structure and function, anemia, impairment of carbohydrate metabolism and the reproductive system, reduced resistance to disease, retarded wound healing, reduced ability to withstand stress, and sudden death.[2]

In humans, similar effects have been reported: dermatitis, inflamed and sore tongue, loss of appetite, nausea, depression, muscle pain, sitophobia (morbid dread of food), pallor, anemia, abnormalities of heart function, burning or prickling sensations, increased sensitivity of the skin, insomnia, extreme lassitude, increased blood levels of cholesterol, and depression of the immune system.

Some of the more subtle metabolic and functional changes may occur sooner, but in experiments in which humans are deprived of biotin and fed a biotin antagonist, the first symptom to appear is usually scaly dermatitis, followed weeks later by pallor, inflammation and atrophy of the tongue, lassitude, sleeplessness, loss of appetite, and evidence of coronary insufficiency. All of these symptoms disappear as soon as 75 to 300 micrograms of biotin are restored to the diet.

Remember, these symptoms are revealed under laboratory conditions in which the subjects are totally deprived of the vitamin. Such total deficiency would be extremely rare. What is more likely to occur is low blood and tissue status of the vitamin—a relatively moderate shortfall between supply and demand, which will nevertheless cause *some* reduction in health.

Many infants suffer seborrheic (greasy, scaling) dermatitis up until the age of six months. *Leiner's Disease* is a similar affliction, only more intense. Because the lesions of these diseases resemble biotin deficiency, many researchers and doctors have successfully used biotin supplementation to clear up the dermatitis. There are almost two dozen reports of biotin having a beneficial effect on both seborrheic dermatitis of infancy and Leiner's Disease.[3] There is also a report of clearing up infantile dermatitis and Leiner's Disease by giving a nursing mother injections of biotin. The babies got enough extra biotin in their mother's milk to correct the deficiency and clear up the dermatitis. Biotin supplements and liver have also had this effect. Since Leiner's Disease appears to be slightly more common in breastfed babies, it would be a good idea if nursing mothers were extra careful to get enough biotin in their diet.[4]

Biotin and Sudden Infant Death Syndrome

A biotin deficiency has been associated with sudden death in animals. Some researchers have attempted to connect a biotin deficiency in newborn infants with SIDS. They point out that SIDS occurs most frequently in the winter months, among male infants, and during the second through fourth months of life, as does biotin-dependent infantile dermatitis. Also, animals which succumb to sudden death generally have a marginal deficiency of biotin. Their death is usually brought on by some stress. SIDS victims have low biotin levels in their liver, and may be subject to some stress, too.[5] No one has tried giving biotin supplements to infants with the symptoms (respiratory distress, apnea) of SIDS. If nothing else, however, these associations give new mothers another reason to be sure their diets are adequate.

Biotin has also been shown to correct certain rare enzymatic deficiencies. In one reported case, a child was "extremely debilitated, shocky, dehydrated," and suffering from a systemic bacterial infection despite the antibiotics he was receiving. The child was given 10 mg. of biotin, orally, and both the symptoms and the biochemical defect disappeared in a matter of hours. The child was well as long as he was maintained on high-dose biotin therapy to correct his enzymatic deficiency.[6] While this particular defect requiring an increased intake of biotin is rare, it does point out that there are too many factors to set one dietary amount that will suffice for all.

HOW MUCH BIOTIN IS ENOUGH?

Nonetheless, the RDA which has been set for biotin is 300 micrograms (.3 mg.) per day for adults and children over four years old. For children under four, the RDA is 150 micrograms.

Some nutritionists maintain that a biotin deficiency can occur only when the biotin in the body is destroyed by an antagonist, such as raw egg white. On the other hand, there is also research which demonstrates that large numbers of people do indeed have low levels of biotin in their blood.[7] These include the elderly, athletes, pregnant women, alcoholics, and people with achlorhydria (absence of hydrochloric acid in the stomach).[8] In pregnant women, for example, the biotin level in the blood starts out lower than in other adults and *decreases* as pregnancy progresses. Biotin in mother's milk after birth, and for at least four days, is too low to be measured. After that, it varies from individual to individual. People with liver disease also have lower than normal levels of biotin.[9] Blood plasma levels of biotin have been shown to drop below normal in children with burns and scalds, too.[10]

Biotin Antagonists

The principal biotin antagonist is *avidin*, a component of raw egg white. Avidin combines with biotin (or *binds* it) and renders the vitamin unavailable for utilization.

A biotin deficiency may also be produced by antibiotics. Researchers believe that bacteria normally found in the intestines can synthesize biotin, which is absorbed into the bloodstream. Antibiotics can kill these bacteria and shut off a potentially important supply of biotin.

TOXICITY

No human or animal experiments have ever demonstrated a toxic reaction to large doses of biotin.

SOURCES OF BIOTIN

Good dietary sources of biotin are liver and other organ meats, egg yolk, peanuts, filberts, mushrooms, and cauliflower. Whole grains are also good sources. Processed cereals and grains, such as white rice and flour, have had most of the biotin removed and none returned through fortification.

Biotin is available in supplement form in doses ranging from a few micrograms up to several hundred micrograms.

9

Pantothenate (Pantothenic Acid)

Imagine yourself standing on a dock in the middle of winter, waiting for the ferry. Your foot slips and the next thing you know you're trying to stay afloat in water that's colder than iced tea. You're too busy to think about it just then, but the amount of pantothenate in your diet could make a difference in whether you make it back to a warm, dry place.

Swimming in cold water is an extreme situation, but the same physiological system which responds to that stress responds to every other stress we encounter. You may never get close enough to cold water to fall in, but do you ever wait for a bus in the middle of winter? Do you ever walk to work or just to the mailbox during a snowstorm? You may live where it's always warm, but do you also live where there are no mental or physical challenges, no problems, no frustrations, no sports, no exercise, no parties, and no work? All of these are stresses. All are common activities most of us cannot avoid and *wouldn't* even if we could. And the body's response to all of them depends on pantothenate.

WHAT PANTOTHENATE DOES

Pantothenate is the essential part of coenzyme A, which is required for cellular metabolism. So *every cell in the body depends on pantothenate*. But, as with other nutrients, there is a particular organ which is especially dependent upon the vitamin: the *adrenal cortex*. This, in part, explains why pantothenate is important to our response to stress, because the adrenal cortex *controls* that response.

When the body is stressed—and this can mean falling in the bay, fighting with your boss, playing tennis, running a marathon, or making love—the adrenal cortex is supposed to secrete hormones which stimulate and maintain the body's reaction to the stress. A whole series of physiological functions have to be rapidly coordinated: blood pressure has to rise, heart rate has to increase, the nervous system and the muscles have to be put on ALERT for action, and the body's mechanism for supplying energy has to be stepped up. Carbohydrate, protein, and fat metabolism have to be mobilized for energy and tissue repair. As far as the body is concerned, the bad words between you and the boss could come to blows. So it prepares for the worst.

The adrenal cortex is the conductor orchestrating all of this activity, and it needs pantothenate in order to do it. How much pantothenate the adrenal cortex needs is determined by how much stress the body must withstand. If more is needed than supplied, the adrenal cortex deteriorates in both structure and function. It starts to hemorrhage, becomes infiltrated with fat, and dies. It doesn't take long for these changes to occur, either, once demand starts to exceed supply. And the more severe the stress, the more severe the damage. Some of the pathological changes are reversible, but if the deficiency has been too severe for too long, the adrenals—and the body's response to stress—are permanently impaired.

The adrenal cortex makes use of cholesterol and vitamin C in orchestrating the body's response to stress. When the adrenal cortex is malfunctioning, vitamin C and cholesterol levels in the gland plummet. Pantothenate can directly affect how far and how fast these substances are depleted, and how quickly they are replaced. During a pantothenate deficiency, vitamin C levels in the adrenal cortex only drop slightly— until the body is stressed, when the vitamin practically *disappears*. The body's excretion of vitamin C also drops during a pantothenate deficiency. The body conserves vitamin C for whatever stress is on the way. (High doses of vitamin C can partially protect against the effects of a pantothenate deficiency.)

The body's response to stress isn't all wrapped up in the adrenal cortex. Energy metabolism, for example, also involves the liver. Levels of glycogen in the liver and sugar in the blood are good indications of the body's response to energy needs during stress. Pantothenate determines how well these levels are maintained.[1] The immune system is also vital to the response to stress. If the immune system weren't part of the overall "beefing up" of the body's functions during stress, we'd get sick every time we worked hard, fought, exercised, played tennis, or made love. Obviously, we do occasionally get sick after periods of stress. When this happens, we say the stress "lowered our resistance." It did just that, but it may not have if the body were getting enough pantothenate. When pantothenate demand exceeds supply, the immune system's production of antibodies falters.[2]

WHAT HAPPENS WHEN PANTOTHENATE DEMAND EXCEEDS SUPPLY

In animals, a pantothenate deficiency produces growth failure, gray hair, degeneration of the testicles, depressed antibody formation, ulcers, fetal abnormalities, deterioration of the cornea, dermatitis, spinal cord deterioration, fatty degeneration of the liver, convulsions, enteritis, coma, hemorrhaging of the kidneys, prolapse of the intestine, and adrenal insufficiency.

The effects of a pantothenate deficiency on people were

revealed in a classic experiment in which four healthy young men were fed a synthetic diet free of pantothenate and injected with known antagonists to the vitamin. Symptoms started to appear during the second week of the deficiency. The men's blood pressure dropped, sometimes so low they would get dizzy when standing up. Their pulse would race after a slight exertion. And they complained of tiredness and slept frequently during the daytime.

During the third week, they complained of constipation and loss of appetite. Personality changes began to occur in the middle of the fourth week. The men grew increasingly quarrelsome, discontented, irritable, and irascible. Numbness and tingling in their hands and feet became increasingly annoying. Their balance, coordination, and reflexes diminished. They came down with respiratory infections one after the other. One man developed pneumonia.

The symptoms were so severe that the doctors decided to give the men pantothenate supplements to overcome the effects of the vitamin antagonists. But the symptoms grew worse. The men grew more fatigued and their sense of well-being deteriorated further. One man suddenly started fits of vomiting. Another became lethargic and slept for an entire day. The doctors were so alarmed by these developments that they stopped the experiment cold, treated the men with cortisone to aid their adrenal glands, restored their regular diet, and gave them multivitamins and injections of the B complex and pantothenate.[3]

CAN EXTRA PANTOTHENATE DO US ANY GOOD?

You might call the deficiencies suffered by these men *heroic*, because they had to go to great lengths to develop them. Though none of us eats a synthetic diet free of the vitamin and receives injections of vitamin antagonists, a marginal deficiency could still make us suffer lesser versions of what they went through. Besides, these men were housed in a practically stress-free environment. They didn't have to cross streets, drive in rush-hour traffic, pay bills, fight with the boss, play handball, or make love. Since pantothenate demand increases during stress, their symptoms would no doubt have occurred *sooner* and been even more severe had they been required to endure stress.

That means we don't necessarily have to eat a pantothenate-free diet and receive injections of vitamin antagonists before we suffer what they did. It also means we might substantially boost our own response to stress if we make sure our pantothenate supply meets the demand. Better performance on the job, on the ski slopes, on the tennis or handball court, and even in bed, could result.

This has been demonstrated in a controlled experiment. Researchers put three groups of rats in cold water and required them to swim until exhaustion. Animals that didn't get the standard requirement of pantothenate were able to swim for only sixteen minutes. Rats fed the standard amount stayed afloat for twenty-nine minutes. But the rats fed "excess" amounts of pantothenate swam for sixty-two minutes—more than twice as long as those on the "adequate" diet. Obviously, the adequate diet wasn't as adequate as the "excess" diet.

The researchers then added two new groups of rats, both groups surgically deprived of their adrenal glands. One group received the standard "adequate" amount of pantothenate, while the other group received pantothenate supplements. The first group was able to swim for nineteen minutes, but the second stayed afloat for thirty-seven minutes. Note that the supplemented animals *with no adrenal glands* swam longer than the animals in the first experiment who still had their glands but received only standard amounts of pantothenate.

The same researchers next tested pantothenate's effect on humans' ability to withstand cold water stress. Volunteers were given 10 grams of pantothenate a day for six weeks, then immersed in cold water. They weren't required to swim until exhaustion, but their body's biochemical response to the stress was measured and compared to that of volunteers who were not given extra pantothenate. All of these measurements indicated that the stress was not taxing the bodies of the supplemented people as much as it was those of the others.[4]

These experiments strongly suggest that getting extra amounts of pantothenate may help us better deal with the stresses we encounter in our lives. The amounts used in the latter experiment were rather high. Although pantothenate is nontoxic, it's impractical to take 10 grams of it every day. More moderate supplementation should have a beneficial effect.

Pantothenate and Arthritis

There appears to be a relationship between pantothenate and arthritis. Some years ago, studies revealed that arthritics have substantially lower blood levels of pantothenate than people without the disease. This alone is not an indication that extra amounts of the vitamin will necessarily help alleviate symptoms. It may only demonstrate that the disease process or the body's response to the disease increases the need for the vitamin. In this case, further studies revealed that as pantothenate levels declined, the symptoms of rheumatoid arthritis grew more frequent and severe.

Several clinical trials followed in which pantothenate was injected intramuscularly in arthritis patients. Some improvement usually followed the therapy, but the improvement was only temporary. In one trial, however, in which the arthritics were also vegetarians, the improvement in the condition and mobility of the joints was more or less permanent. Only one out of ten patients returned with recurrence of symptoms within fifteen months. This suggests that there may be additional metabolic factors besides blood level of pantothenate, and that vegetarians may be able to take better advantage of them.[5]

Pantothenate and Ulcerative Colitis

One of the characteristics of pantothenate deficiency is

ulceration of the intestine. When such lesions in the intestines of pantothenate-deficient animals have been examined, they are similar to those seen in human ulcerative colitis. This has led researchers to suggest that pantothenate plays a role in this disease. The first step in any such investigation is to test pantothenate levels in the blood of people with the disease. Such tests reveal no differences. However, when the level of *metabolically active* pantothenate (coenzyme A) in the intestinal tissue is measured, people with ulcerative colitis have much lower levels than people without the disease.

This suggests that people with the disease have a *metabolic defect* which inhibits the conversion of pantothenate to its active form *at the site of the lesion*. The logical next step would be to test the effects of pantothenate supplements on people with the disease.[6]

Pantothenate Speeds Healing

Pantothenate helps surgical patients recover quicker. One group of fifty surgical patients were given 500 mg. of the vitamin on the day of their surgery (abdominal) and for five days afterwards. They healed and recovered quicker, had less nausea, and were generally better off than another group of fifty similar patients not given pantothenate supplements.[7]

Pantothenate, Radiation, and Allergies

One stress we should all worry about in this age of nuclear power plant accidents is radiation. A Hungarian study found that pantothenate supplements prolonged the survival of mice exposed to lethal radiation by two hundred percent. This same Hungarian researcher found that pantothenate supplements diminished the severity of the skin's reaction when exposed to an allergen.[8] One of the legendary uses of pantothenate is in the reduction of allergies.

Does Pantothenate Prolong Life?

A lot of people wonder whether vitamins, or a particular

vitamin, can *prolong life*. Such experiments are rare, since most researchers prefer to concentrate on one specific function which affects health, and where the factors are relatively limited—rather than on the length of life, where the factors are immensely complicated. Nonetheless, a venturesome researcher will now and then take a stab at finding out how a particular nutrient, or combination of nutrients, affects life-span. Most scientists shy away from experiments in which it is practically impossible to separate factors and explain why *this* happened or why *that* didn't. That, of course, doesn't mean these studies have no value for us, who merely want some ideas on how to live healthier, and perhaps longer, lives.

One researcher who carried out such an experiment with pantothenate was Roger Williams, the first scientist to identify, isolate, and synthesize pantothenate. Dr. Williams fed one group of mice a diet containing "adequate" pantothenate and another group of mice "extra" pantothenate. The mice who got adequate pantothenate lived an average of 550 days, while the supplemented group lived an average of 653 days, or nineteen percent longer. Dr. Williams does not explain these results by claiming that pantothenate is a miracle substance. Rather, he concludes that some of the mice had increased requirements for the vitamin, and that these requirements were satisfied in the supplemented group and not satisfied in the other group. Again, what is "adequate" for one is not necessarily adequate for all.[9]

HOW MUCH PANTOTHENATE DO WE NEED?

The RDA for pantothenate ranges from 5 mg. to 10 mg. for adults. Once more, the RDA is an arbitrary figure and one should not place too much faith in it.

Pantothenate levels drop during pregnancy, indicating an increased need. So pregnant women should be very carful about getting enough. Low salt diets also seem to raise the requirement for pantothenate, since animals on a low salt diet suffer the symptoms of a pantothenate deficiency more severely. A low-protein diet stresses the adrenals and raises the pantothenate requirement, too.[10]

Folate and biotin are necessary for the proper utilization of pantothenate, so a deficiency in either of these will increase requirements for pantothenate. Supplements of either biotin or pantothenate will lessen the symptoms of a deficiency of the other. Antibiotics may also raise requirements by destroying bacteria in the gut which synthesize the vitamin.

Any stress will increase requirements for pantothenate. This does not necessarily mean that supplementation is necessary. But it does mean that people who undergo stress—and who doesn't?—should ask themselves if they're satisfied with their response to stress and then doublecheck their diet to see if their pantothenate status is what it should be.

TOXICITY

Pantothenate is relatively nontoxic. No researcher has ever succeeded in producing toxic symptoms in people. In animals, however, doses of over 2 to 3 grams per kilogram of body weight are lethal. It would probably take daily doses in excess of 7 grams over very long periods of time to produce toxicity (liver impairment) in people.[11]

SOURCES OF PANTOTHENATE

Pantothenate, as its name implies, is found just about everywhere in plant and animal tissues, in varying amounts. The best sources are organ meats, egg yolk, peanuts, broccoli, cauliflower, cabbage, whole grains, and bran. Fair sources are meat, milk, and fruits. The richest natural source is royal jelly, the substance worker bees feed to the queen bee.

Processing, canning, and freezing result in considerable losses of pantothenate. One should not rely on processed foods for an adequate supply of pantothenate. Pantothenate is not ordinarily destroyed by cooking; however, exposure to acids and alkalies will destroy it.

Pantothenate supplements are available in a wide range of doses, from a few milligrams to several hundred milligrams.

10

Choline

Choline's status as a vitamin is somewhat nebulous. It does occur in many foods along with other B complex factors, and it does seem to be a required dietary factor in the growth and development of several species of animals. A choline deficiency in the rat produces fatty liver and hemorrhaging kidneys. And choline/cobalamin-deprived mice suffer a depression of the immune response.

But opposition to choline's identity as a vitamin arises because it apparently can be synthesized in the body from the amino acid *methionine*. And choline is found in the body in such large amounts, it may be a structural component rather than a catalyst of essential metabolic reactions.

These two facts may not be enough to disqualify choline as a vitamin. Niacin can be synthesized in the body if adequate tryptophan is supplied, yet no one talks about disqualifying niacin as a vitamin. Furthermore, recent research indicates that there are conditions in which the body does not synthesize an "adequate" amount of choline for all its needs. In addition, dietary choline has recently been shown to affect choline levels at various key points in the body. While neither of these proves choline is a vitamin, remember the term *vitamin* is quite arbitrary and that there is often as much economics and politics behind a substance's definition as a vitamin as there is science.

WHAT CHOLINE DOES

For the purposes of this book, choline is a vitamin because dietary levels can, according to reliable research, affect health. Choline has been shown to be helpful in the treatment of several neurological disorders, including tardive dyskinesia, Huntington's Disease, Gilles de la Tourette's Disease, Friedreich's Ataxia, presenile dementia, manic-depression, and Alzheimer's Disease.[1] We'll look at choline's role in some of these, and also how it may play a role in heart disease and cancer.

Choline and Tardive Dyskinesia

Choline's role in neurological diseases begins with its role in *normal* neurological function. Choline is a component of *acetylcholine*, a neurotransmitter. When a nerve impulse jumps the gap from one neuron to another, a neurotransmitter must be there. Don't lose the significance of that reaction in its apparent simplicity. Everything we do depends on those nerve impulses.

Tardive dyskinesia results when some of those impulses are deranged by certain drugs commonly given to psychotic patients (haloperidol and phenothiazine). This derangement results in a grotesque loss of control over the facial muscles. Involuntary grimaces, chewing, puckering, and tongue protrusions result. Until a few years ago, nothing could be done for people suffering this man-made, or iatrogenic (doctor-induced), disease—except to take their drugs away, which usually resulted in worse mental symptoms *in addition* to lingering tardive dyskinesia.

Doctors then theorized that tardive dyskinesia resulted from the drug's interference with the neurotransmitter acetylcholine. Simultaneous research indicated that dietary choline could affect brain levels of acetylcholine in animals. The next step involved a leap of faith in science. Doctors tried boosting human brain levels of acetylcholine by giving high doses of choline to people with tardive dyskinesia. While no one has volunteered to have his brain dissected to measure acetylcholine levels, high doses of choline did have a beneficial effect on tardive dyskinesia. In one study, massive doses of choline (150 mg. per kilogram of body weight daily the first week, 200 mg./kg. thereafter) were given orally to twenty psychiatric patients also suffering tardive dyskinesia. The spasms decreased in nine people, worsened in one, and were unchanged in ten. This is a strikingly better track record than any other treatment. Choline did not interfere with the therapeutic effects of the psychiatric drugs. Other trials with choline have had similar, or even better results. Many of the patients in the above study were elderly and had been receiving drugs for many years. Doctors speculate that the choline may not have been able to overcome all the effects of the drugs because of how long the people had been taking them.[2]

Choline and Memory

Alzheimer's Disease is another name for presenile dementia. The first symptom is usually memory loss. Researchers believe that the nerve cells that perform memory functions use acetylcholine. If this is so, boosting dietary choline should also boost acetylcholine concentractions and improve memory. Several studies have tried supplementary choline on people with Alzheimer's Disease, and the results are encouraging. In one study, memory was measurably improved after three weeks of choline therapy. Relatives of the patients, and the patients themselves, reported that the improvement was substantial.[3] In another study, both doctors and nurses observed changes in elderly people given supplementary choline (5 to 10 grams per day) for their Alzheimer's disease. The patients were "less irritable, more aware of their surroundings," and able to find their way around the building again.[4]

If choline can improve the memories of people with Alzheimer's Disease, can it do the same or better for normal, healthy people? Apparently it can. College students and recent graduates were given a single oral dose of choline (10 grams) and tested on two forms of memory tests, "serial learning" and "selective reminding." Choline decreased substantially the time it took for the subjects to master a fixed sequence of unrelated words (serial learning), and significantly improved their recall of low imagery words (selective reminding).[5] In another study, choline slightly and temporarily improved intellectual functioning in twelve healthy, young subjects.[6]

Huntington's Chorea, or Huntington's Disease, is similar to tardive dyskinesia in that the sufferer loses control over certain muscles. Unlike tardive dyskinesia, however, it is not brought on by drugs, and dementia usually occurs along with the spasms. Choline has been tried in the treatment of this disease with enough encouraging results to warrant further study, but not with the degree of success found in tardive dyskinesia.[7]

Choline is finding more and more potential applications in the treatment of diseases of the nervous system. Research in Europe has found the vitamin useful in the treatment of depressive diseases. In eight psychiatric patients suffering from a range of symptoms, including hypochondria, depression, sleeplessness, paranoia, suicidal tendencies, anxiety, and moodiness, choline injections resulted in significant improvement in all the patients. The most consistent effect was the complete disappearance of depression in all patients.[8]

Although no serious side effects resulted from the use of choline in high doses in any of these treatments, the nature of the diseases themselves are such that they would normally be treated by a physician. It is interesting to speculate whether smaller doses of choline might not help people who were not yet ill enough to need a doctor's care. No research has been done in that area.

Choline and Heart Disease

Animal experiments have shown that a diet deficient in choline and high in fat produces cardiovascular lesions, whereas the same diet supplemented with choline does not. Further experiments have shown that choline supplementation also protects animals against a high-fat diet combined with toxic doses of vitamin D (which also produces cardiovascular lesions).[9] The effect of supplementary choline on heart disease mortality in people was tested by giving one group of 115 heart patients choline supplements and another equal group none or a placebo. Within three years there were 30 deaths among the unsupplemented group and 12 deaths among the supplemented group.[10] The results of both these studies are remarkable, but again, don't be tempted by the interpretation that a single vitamin is the answer to heart disease. Both of these studies were performed more than twenty-five years ago, and a search of the literature indicates that the thread of this research was never continued.

Choline and Protection of the Liver

Rats fed a choline-deficient diet developed liver tumors when fed a cancer-causing chemical. However, rats fed a choline-supplemented or choline-adequate diet developed no tumors when they were fed *larger amounts* of the carcinogen.[11] This study suggests that choline does have a role as a "vitamin," since all that the organism needs is not supplied by either the diet or internal synthesis. Whether choline might provide a useful treatment for cancer has not in any way been tested. It is a reasonable assumption, however, that choline "adequacy" in the body plays a role in our defenses against cancer and that a deficiency might in some way compromise

our defense. This much is true, of course, for many other
nutrients as well.

REQUIREMENTS, SOURCES,
AND TOXICITY OF CHOLINE

No RDA for choline has been set. Average diets have been
found to contain from 250 mg. to 600 mg. Of course, this is
no indication of what is "adequate."

The best natural source of choline is lecithin. Some of the
above-mentioned studies used lecithin as a source of choline.
Other sources of B vitamins, such as whole grains, yeast, fish,
eggs, legumes, and liver are also good sources of choline.

Choline supplements are available in a wide range of doses,
from a few milligrams to several hundred milligrams. Some
choline supplements have the drawback that they are degraded
by the gut bacteria and produce a substance which causes a
fishy odor. Lecithin does not cause this problem, since it is
absorbed by the intestine. However, lecithin does have the
disadvantage of supplying a considerable number of calories.

Choline is relatively nontoxic. At the high doses used in
some of the psychiatric experiments (for tardive dyskinesia),
nausea, abdominal cramps, and diarrhea were suffered by a
few patients. Also, a small number of psychiatric patients
became depressed when given choline.

11

Inositol

Inositol is another B complex factor with nebulous status. Animal experiments have identified it as a necessary factor for growth and survival, but there has been little human research on specific deficiency symptoms. Inositol is concentrated in the skeletal and heart muscles, lungs, liver, brain, blood, milk, urine, and eggs. Its metabolic role in these and other tissues is not yet known.

Nonetheless, some research has indicated possible practical uses for inositol. Animal experiments have demonstrated that raising dietary inositol levels prevents the decrease in motor nerve conduction that results from degeneration of nerve insulation in diabetes. Inositol supplementation in the diets of human diabetics had a similar effect. The more inositol in the diet (maximum 1400 mg.), the better the nerve conduction.

When the people ate an inositol-deficient diet, nerve conduction was lowest. An inositol-"adequate" diet improved nerve conduction over the deficient diet, but not as much as the supplemented diet.[1]

Inositol has also been shown to be of possible use against some forms of cancer. Intravenous injections of inositol inhibited tumor growth in mice, in one experiment. The degree of inhibition increased with the amount of inositol used. One doctor tried high doses of inositol (3 to 4 grams daily) in people with advanced cases of cancer of the genitourinary tract. The seven cases with terminal malignancies of the prostate, penis, and testicle were not apparently benefited. But six cases of bladder cancer were helped. Their tumors reduced in size, and their hematuria (blood in the urine) disappeared.[2]

Inositol has also been shown to increase the ability of the liver to resist fatty infiltration and damage by toxins. It has also been reported to lower cholesterol in man and animals. However, the source of the inositol was lecithin. Since lecithin also contains choline and other substances, the cholesterol-lowering effect may not have been due to inositol alone, even though the researchers did attribute the effect to inositol.[3]

REQUIREMENTS, SOURCES, AND TOXICITY OF INOSITOL

No RDA for inositol has been set. An average diet supplies about one gram per day. Apparently, intestinal flora (bacteria) can synthesize a certain amount of inositol which is made available to the body. Sources of inositol include lecithin, yeast, organ meats, nuts, fruit, vegetables, and whole grains. Inositol supplements are available in a wide range of doses, from less than a hundred milligrams up to several hundred. The fact that both animals and people have been aided by supplements of inositol indicates that the body does not always synthesize an "adequate" amount.

There are no reports of toxic reactions to inositol.

12

PABA

PABA, or para-aminobenzoic acid, like choline and inositol, has not yet been "officially" recognized as a vitamin. Such recognition usually means that the evidence in favor of a substance's essentiality is *so* overwhelming that the government is more willing to bear the wrath of the food industry than it is the weight of scientific evidence. When a nutrient is recognized as "essential," pressure is immediately placed on the food industry because food processing *removes* most nutrients. Naturally, the fewer nutrients that are recognized as essential, the fewer the industry will have to either replace or list on the label as nonexistent. Since the food industry has one of the most powerful lobbies in Washington, evidence in favor of a nutrient's essentiality must be incredibly overwhelming.

The evidence in favor of PABA's essentiality is nowhere near overwhelming enough, and probably won't be for some time. Nonetheless, it is tentatively identified as a vitamin because a PABA deficiency in rats produces gray hair. Deficiencies of pantothenate, biotin, and folate produce gray hair in rats, too. But PABA has achieved somewhat of a reputation as the anti-gray hair vitamin." No known controlled studies have demonstrated that PABA is of practical use in preventing gray hair in people. Yet there have been individual reports of massive doses of PABA darkening the hair.

PABA is also necessary for growth and survival of chicks.

The most common use of PABA is as a *sunscreen*. In solution (usually alcohol), PABA *applied to the skin* is the most effective sunscreen available. A sunscreen has the ability to screen out harmful portions of the ultraviolet light, those that cause sunburn and cancer. A sunshade merely blocks all the sun's rays. PABA has been shown to protect animals almost completely from the cancer-causing effects of ultraviolet light, even when they were also treated with a substance that becomes highly carcinogenic when exposed to ultraviolet light.[1]

Skin cancer is the single most common form of cancer. Over 300,000 cases of skin cancer develop each year, 5000 of which are eventually fatal. Sunburn is also a factor in aging, and many doctors advise avoiding the sun as much as possible. For people who can't or won't stay out of the sun, PABA is a must.

PABA has been used in oral doses ranging from 12 to 24 grams per day in the treatment of many skin diseases, including fibrotic skin diseases and *pemphigus, Peyronie's Disease, reticulum cell sarcoma,* and *scleroderma*. Doses of 1 to 4 grams, taken every two to three hours, produced a good response in seven out of ten people with *chronic discoid lupus erythematosus*.

PABA was once used in the treatment of *rickettsial* (denotes the type of organism) infections, including typhus and Rocky Mountain Spotted Fever. Of course, with the development of antibiotics, PABA was no longer used.

PABA has been shown to have a protective effect against ozone. Rats injected with PABA better survive the effects of ozone exposure. Human red blood cells also are protected from ozone by PABA. These effects are most likely attributable to PABA's antioxidant properties. PABA taken orally has also been shown to decrease the toxicity of arsenic and antimony.[2]

REQUIREMENTS, SOURCES, AND TOXICITY OF PABA

No RDA has been set for PABA. Natural sources include yeast, liver, and other B vitamin sources. Supplements of PABA are available in amounts ranging from a few milligrams to several hundred milligrams. PABA is generally considered nontoxic to people. The vitamin should not be given in supplemental form at the same time as sulfa drugs, since PABA deactivates the drugs. Fatty changes in the liver, kidneys, and heart have been reported in a small number of people taking extremely large doses of PABA for extended periods of time.

13

Vitamin C

Several thousand years ago, people were exiled from a nutritional Garden of Eden: the human body somehow lost the ability to make its own vitamin C. As a result of this genetic misstep—which also affected monkeys, guinea pigs, a certain fruit-eating bat that lives in India, and the Bulbul bird—many millions of people now spend many millions of dollars on many billions of milligrams of vitamin C. All are dutifully swallowed in hopes of avoiding a range of diseases and maladies wide enough to boggle the mind of all but the most daring snake oil salesman: the common cold, flu, infections, back trouble, heart disease, mental illness, arthritis, infertility, slow healing, fatigue, heat and cold stress, diabetes, bone disease, the toxic effects of pollutants, and cancer.

A random telephone survey a few years ago discovered that out of the hundred people called, sixty-seven were taking vitamin C supplements.[1]

Are these people all wasting their money? Is excess intake of

125

vitamin C merely contributing to what some have called "the most expensive urine in the world?" What, exactly, *does* vitamin C do? Does it really do the things a lot of people claim it does?

Let's start with the basics before describing some of the fascinating research that's been done on vitamin C. And there is a *lot* of research! Whenever a doctor, nutritionist, or writer pooh-poohs something about vitamin C with the statement, "There's no evidence," you know he or she hasn't kept up with the scientific literature. For vitamin C is one of the most heavily researched and "published about" substances in scientific and medical journals.

WHAT VITAMIN C DOES

Vitamin C, or ascorbic acid, has many vital functions within the body. It has a role in the metabolism of amino acids, most likely as a coenzyme. It facilitates the conversion of folic acid (folate) to its active form, folinic acid. Vitamin C also has a vital part in cellular respiration. But by far the most well-known role of vitamin C is its essentiality in the formation of collagen and other fibrous tissue. Collagen is the main supportive protein of skin, tendon, bone, teeth, cartilage, and connective tissue. The structural and functional integrity of capillary walls depends on vitamin C. Whenever tissue has to grow, develop, or repair itself after injury, a collagenous intracellular matrix must be set down to hold everything together. If vitamin C is not present in adequate quantities, this matrix is not set down, or it is incompletely constructed. A prolonged deficiency of the vitamin will deteriorate structures already present. So just about all the tissues in the body depend on vitamin C for proper growth, development, and maintenance.

Vitamin C is absorbed from the small intestine, circulated in the blood, and stored in the tissues. The adrenals, pituitary gland, thymus, and corpus luteum contain higher amounts than other tissue. Metabolically active tissue also contains higher than normal amounts.

Vitamin C concentrations are usually highest in the adrenal glands. When the organism is stressed in any way, vitamin C is mobilized from the glands, as well as from other tissues, and higher amounts of it appear in the urine. This is an indication that vitamin C plays an important role in the body's ability to withstand stress. Vitamin A-deficient rats lose the ability to synthesize vitamin C, and their adrenal glands malfunction. Vitamin C supplementation restores normal adrenal function, however.[2] In humans, many of the symptoms of vitamin C deficiency (scurvy) are identical to those of adrenal insufficiency: fatigue, muscle weakness, digestive disorders, and reduced ability to tolerate stress.[3]

Vitamin C is also an antioxidant, which means it helps protect cells and tissues from damaging oxidation. This fact alone could account for vitamin C's usefulness in the treatment of many diseases, since researchers are finding out more and more how really large a role oxidation plays in the disease process.[4] Stimulation of muscle tissue raises the tissue requirements for vitamin C, because exercised muscle uses the vitamin at an increased rate.[5] This may, in part, explain why vitamin C deficiency produces muscle weakness.

WHAT HAPPENS WHEN VITAMIN C DEMAND EXCEEDS SUPPLY

The first lesions of vitamin C deficiency (scurvy) result from the breakdown in the intracellular matrix which, quite literally, holds the body together. Among the first symptoms are hemorrhaging, delayed healing of traumatized soft tissue and broken bones, generalized swelling, inflammation of the gums, loosening of the teeth, separation of the ends of the long bones, emaciation, and swollen joints. Anemia, weakness, weight loss, irritability, aches and pains in the joints, extremities and muscles, easy bruising and bleeding, swelling and hardening of the hair follicles, drying of the tear glands, hypochondria, hysteria, depression, and other neurological disturbances, can also occur. Infantile scurvy includes most of these symptoms, plus impaired growth and development.

Most schoolchildren learn that scurvy was the scourge of the British Navy until James Lind discovered that the juice of citrus fruit would completely prevent it. What we often don't learn is that Lind's advice was not taken until *forty years after* he gave it and demonstrated its effectiveness. Scurvy was widespread among groups of people such as sailors and soldiers who had to subsist without fresh food for long periods of time. Even after Lind's discovery was accepted by his fellow British physicians, it was many decades before the knowledge spread very far. As many as fifteen percent of the deaths in the American Civil War have been attributed to scurvy, and that was more than a hundred years after Lind's work.

The RDA of vitamin C is based on the amount it takes to prevent the frank appearance of the above-described symptoms. Many doctors and nutritionists today believe that *subclinical scurvy*—a deficit between what the body needs of vitamin C and what it gets, too small to result in gross symptomatology, yet large enough to cause chronic damage and illness—is rampant. This bears upon the question of how much vitamin C we actually need in our diet. But for now, keep two things about scurvy in mind: the wide range of symptoms and the forty years it took for James Lind to convince the medical establishment that such a horrible disease could be caused by such a simple gap in the diet.

Vitamin C and Fertility

Japanese doctors tried giving 400 mg. of vitamin C to forty-two infertile women they had been unsuccessfully treating with a fertility drug (clomiphene). Vitamin C alone enabled fourteen percent of the women to ovulate. However, when vitamin C was added to the drug treatment, forty percent of the women began to ovulate, and twenty-one percent later became pregnant. The ovary is one of the sites in the body where vitamin C is concentrated.[6] A study of women who gave birth to babies with central nervous system defects found that these women had lower than normal levels of vitamin C in their bodies.[7]

Heat and Cold Stress

South African doctors found that mine workers' vitamin C stores dropped during their first few months of working in the hot, humid mines, so they conducted a test to see if supplemental vitamin C would help the workers adjust to the stress. New mine workers were given either a vitamin C supplement (250 to 500 mg.) or a placebo pill, and observed while they worked in a controlled climate chamber designed to acclimate workers to mine conditions. Vitamin C definitely helped them adjust to the heat, since the body temperatures of the supplemented workers were lower than the others' on every day of the test. After four days in the heat, thirty-five percent of the supplemented workers were fully accustomed to the heat, whereas only five percent of the unsupplemented workers were.[8]

Vitamin C also helps us deal with cold stress. In one experiment, three groups of guinea pigs (which don't manufacture their own vitamin C) were given either deficient, adequate, or "excessive" amounts of vitamin C in their diet, and then exposed to severe cold (minus ten degrees centigrade for fifty-five minutes). Whereas recovery was slow in the deficient and "adequate" groups, and some animals died, the "excessive" group recovered rapidly and completely.[9] Interestingly, this study was performed to find out if vitamin C *impaired* the response to stress!

Vitamin C and Healing

Because vitamin C is necessary for the production of collagen and the laying down of the intracellular matrix, it's not difficult to understand how important it is to the healing process. No one questions the fact that a vitamin C deficiency will slow healing. But what can *extra* vitamin C do for people who already have an "adequate" amount?

Several studies have demonstrated that "excessive" amounts of vitamin C can actually *speed up the healing process* in comparison to people or animals with "adequate" levels. In one of these studies, ten surgical patients with pressure ulcers were given 500 mg. of vitamin C twice a day, and ten were given a placebo. All twenty had normal and more or less equal blood levels of the vitamin before the supplementation began. The rate of healing was measured in both groups for a month. The vitamin C-supplemented group's healing rate was seventy percent faster than the placebo group's on a weekly basis, and after a month the mean reduction in the size of the ulcers was almost twice as great in the supplemented group.[10]

Several animal studies have demonstrated the difference between "adequate" vitamin C intake and "enough to help wounds heal faster." In one study, the strength in healing wounds of guinea pigs was found to be proportional to the amount of vitamin C in the diet.[11] In another study, rabbits injected with vitamin C healed more completely and without corneal perforation after alkali burns in the eyes. Unsupplemented rabbits suffered slow healing and numerous perforations. This study is significant in that even though rabbits synthesize their own vitamin C, levels of the vitamin in the aqueous humor dropped and remained low after the burns.[12] Apparently, a severe stress or trauma can create *localized vitamin C deficiencies* in the tissue bearing the brunt of the stress.

Paraplegic patients with pressure sores were measured and found to have "normal" levels of vitamin C. Nonetheless, when they were given 1 gram of vitamin C per day, their collagen production was boosted. Other studies in which vitamin C levels were measured in people indicate that after surgery, tissue levels of the vitamin drop by as much as forty-two percent. On the basis of such evidence, many doctors and nutritionists recommend supplements of vitamin C for people undergoing surgery or some other process that requires healing.[13] Unfortunately, most doctors are unaware of or resist this advice, and many hospital patients are needlessly endangered;

one study found blood levels of vitamin C low enough to indicate *scurvy* in *all 1400* surgical patients with infections that were tested! The researchers did not hazard a guess as to whether the infections were an early indication of scurvy.[14]

There are many common, if less dangerous, situations in which vitamin C can help the body heal faster or better. A Navy physician found that 600 mg. of vitamin C (plus 600 mg. of bioflavonoid complex—see chapter on bioflavonoids) cut the healing time for herpes sores on the lips to *less than half* when the treatment was begun at the first signs of the infection.[15] Vitamin C supplements (1000 mg.) have been shown to speed the healing of stubborn prickly heat rash, too.[16]

Low back pain can also respond to large daily supplements of vitamin C. Texas neurosurgeon James Greenwood has been using doses in excess of 1000 mg. per day on hundreds of people with degeneration of the discs in the lower back. Vitamin C apparently helps the disc connective tissue strengthen and heal. Many of his patients have been able to completely avoid surgery after vitamin C treatment. He also reports that 1000 mg. of vitamin C per day helps *prevent* back trouble.[17]

One thing to keep in mind here is that deterioration of a structure like the connective tissue of the back can occur for many reasons. Lack of exercise can contribute, too. In fact, when a muscle or structural component suffers from underuse, the nutritional supply to that part is often impaired, which, of course, can lead to further deterioration. This suggests that people who cannot help being immobile, such as hospital patients, should increase their supply of certain vitamins and minerals, but that people who can exercise should do so and not rely on supplements alone to keep their bodies well.

Vitamin C and Cardiovascular Disease

Evidence has been mounting for decades that vitamin C plays an important role in heart disease. For at least eight weeks after a heart attack, for example, white blood cell levels of the vitamin fall to the levels found in scurvy. This indicates that heart disease patients need more vitamin C after an attack.[18] But there's plenty of evidence that vitamin C levels *can help decide whether that attack will ever come.* More than a quarter century ago, it was demonstrated that vitamin C deficiency in guinea pigs produced atherosclerotic lesions that were identical to those of the human disease. And injections of high doses of vitamin C appeared to partially protect animals fed a high cholesterol diet.[19] The same researchers subsequently measured vitamin C levels in human arteries, and found that arteries with atherosclerotic lesions had much lower levels of vitamin C than arteries free of lesions.[20]

The implication of these studies is that a localized deficiency first allows the ground substance of the blood vessels to deteriorate, and then causes the deposit of cholesterol plaques.

Several studies have shown that vitamin C lowers blood cholesterol and triglycerides. Early Russian studies reveal that as little as 500 mg. twice a day, a low-fat diet, abstention from alcohol, and a moderate amount of exercise lowered cholesterol as much as fifty percent and alleviated many of the symptoms of heart disease. Blood pressure dropped to normal in many patients, and they subsequently could return to a normal life.[21] These Russian studies were performed in the early 1950s. More than twenty years later, Czechoslovakian doctors gave 1 gram supplements twice a day to eighty-two men and women between the ages of fifty and seventy-five. They found that vitamin C did, in fact, lower blood levels of cholesterol, but that the degree of lowering was dependent on how high the levels were in the first place. Persons with low cholesterol levels experienced little or no lowering. In some people with low cholesterol (below 200 mg.), vitamin C appeared to slightly *raise* their levels. However, in people with cholesterol levels above 230 mg. , vitamin C produced a substantial decline in sixty percent of the patients, a decline which persisted for nine months while the experiment was still proceeding and for six weeks after the supplements stopped. The researchers concluded that "chronic, latent vitamin C deficiency" produced the high blood levels of cholesterol.[22] And American researchers have succeeded in lowering triglyceride levels from fifty to seventy percent in heart patients,[23] and lowering blood cholesterol in rabbits fed a high cholesterol diet.[24]

In one study, no supplemental vitamin C was given, but blood levels of vitamin C, cholesterol and triglycerides were measured in 600 fasting blood donors aged twenty-five to fifty-five (half male, half female). For both sexes, the lower their blood levels of vitamin C, the higher were their cholesterol and triglycerides. Normal blood levels of cholesterol and triglycerides were most common in the group with a high vitamin C concentration. In fact, a person with high vitamin C levels was *two to three times* less likely to have high blood fats.[25]

A British study found that high blood levels of vitamin C were associated with high levels of HDL cholesterol. (HDL, or high density lipoprotein, contains cholesterol that is on its way *out* of the body. LDL, or low density lipoprotein, contains cholesterol on its way *into* the cells, including those lining the arteries. A high HDL cholesterol level is a good thing to have.) Some subjects in the study were found to respond to vitamin C supplementation with higher HDL levels, and in one man, a respiratory infection brought about a drop in both vitamin C levels and HDL levels.[26]

Vitamin C also helps protect against cardiovascular disease by means of its role in the clotting of blood. One of the primary dangers in cardiovascular disease is that blood clots will form when and where they're least required—in blood vessels narrowed by atherosclerotic plaques. Such a clot, or *thrombus*, can cut off or decrease the blood supply to the heart, brain, or some other organ, and result in disability or death. Several studies have shown that vitamin C inhibits or prolongs the process of *platelet aggregation*, in which blood platelets group together to form clots.[27] And another study demonstrated 1 gram of supplemental vitamin C substantially increased fibrinolytic activity (which prevents clots from forming), even when dietary fat was increased.[28]

Vitamin C affects the strength of the small blood vessels, the capillaries, as it does the arteries. One of the symptoms of scurvy which James Lind noted was "varicose veins under the tongue." Some doctors have noted the same vascular changes under the tongues of people with low vitamin C levels. And just as the initial lesion in atherosclerosis is thought to be the deterioration of the artery wall, the initial lesion in cerebro-vascular disease may be hemorrhages in the tiny blood vessels that feed the brain. High blood pressure, of course, raises the danger that such hemorrhages will occur more frequently and eventually strike a major capillary and cause death or severe disability. Since low vitamin C levels have been found in persons with capillary fragility, and since one of vitamin C's functions is to maintain the integrity of the blood vessels, it's reasonable to assume that a diet high in vitamin C will afford some increased degree of protection from stroke and other forms of cerebrovascular disease.[29]

The "bottom line" question people ask is whether supple-mental vitamin C will offer complete protection from cardio-vascular disease. What this question really asks is whether it's possible to take enough vitamin C to overcome the effects of a high-fat diet and a low-exercise lifestyle. Even though studies with rabbits have demonstrated that large doses of vitamin C (injected) substantially inhibited the deposit of atherosclerotic plaque in the arteries of rabbits fed a high-cholesterol diet,[30] the inclination is to answer *"No."* The real question should be whether a high vitamin C diet, with or without supple-mentation, will *contribute* to the prevention and treatment of cardiovascular disease. The answer to that, based on the evidence, seems to be *"Of course."* But don't expect vitamin C to make up for a refusal to acknowledge all the *other* evidence of what helps people avoid heart and blood vessel disease.

Vitamin C and Diabetes

Diabetics in general, and insulin-dependent diabetics in particular, have been found to have lower-than-normal levels of vitamin C in their blood.[31] This apparent lack of, or increased need for, vitamin C may result in some of the disabling side effects of diabetes. For example, diabetics with high blood levels of cholesterol also tend to have low blood levels of vitamin C. Giving 500 mg. supplements of vitamin C daily to these people resulted in a "striking decline" in high blood cholesterol and a moderate decline in triglycerides. The doctors who carried out this study concluded that vitamin C supplements corrected the local tissue's vitamin deficiency, and improved the liver's ability to metabolize cholesterol into harmless by-products.[32]

Diabetics frequently suffer the effects of increased capillary fragility: easy bruising and bleeding. When the diabetic's diet contains *normal* amounts of vitamin C, capillary strength is not increased. However, supplements of 1 gram of vitamin C restore capillary strength to normal.[33]

Another researcher has suggested that supplements of vitamin C could help prevent cataracts in diabetics. Animal experiments (guinea pigs) have demonstrated that cataracts develop predominantly in diabetic animals fed a vitamin C-deficient diet.[34]

Vitamin C and Infection

One of the most controversial issues involving vitamin C is whether it has any effect on the frequency or severity of colds. Responding to claims by Linus Pauling that a regular supplement of 1000 mg. (1 gram) of vitamin C would significantly reduce the number of colds and days of illness, a Canadian epidemiologist, Terence Anderson, M.D., Ph.D., set out to *disprove* that vitamin C could do any good for cold sufferers. Dr. Anderson put over 800 people on either 1 gram daily of vitamin C or a placebo. During the first three days of any illness, the volunteers were required to quadruple the dose. Frequency of illness, total days of illness, and number of days of disability (confined to house) were measured and compared. After fourteen weeks, the vitamin C group had seven percent fewer episodes of illness and twelve percent fewer days of illness. These differences were judged to be not statistically significant, considering the number of people involved in the study. However, one difference was significant: the amount of *disability* suffered by the vitamin C group was thirty percent less than that of the other group.

Dr. Anderson attempted a second trial, involving 3500 volunteers. But certain factors disqualified the results of that study. A third trial, however, confirmed the results of the first. Using slightly *lower* doses of vitamin C, people achieved a twenty-five percent reduction in the days of disability because of cold symptoms.[35]

Dr. Anderson's experiments do not prove that vitamin C actually *prevents* colds. But they do demonstrate that vitamin C has undeniable benefit for people with colds, and that the vitamin helps the body fight off colds.

How does vitamin C help fight infections? Several studies have demonstrated a whole range of effects on the immune system. White blood cell levels of vitamin C are known to fall during stress. That stress can include a heart attack, an infection, or simply overwork. Adding extra vitamin C to the diet raises the white blood cell levels back to, and even beyond, normal.[36] Vitamin C has also been shown to boost the activity of the lymphocytes, which are the white blood cells responsible for resisting infecting organisms.[37] Vitamin C has been shown in several studies to reverse the depression of the immune system by steroid drugs.[38]

Vitamin C also boosts the body's production of a natural antibacterial, antiviral substance called *interferon*. Interferon is especially efficient against viruses. If cells attacked by a virus can produce enough interferon, the virus will be prevented from reproducing and the infection will be successfully resisted. Interferon also stimulates at least one other member of the infection-fighting team, the *macrophages*, which are large cells whose special function is to devour any invading cell, whether it's a virus, bacterium, or cancer cell. Vitamin C's positive effect on interferon production also has encouraging implications for fighting cancer.[39]

Back as far as the 1930s, vitamin C's effect on the body's resistance to infection was known and studied. In 1935, very high blood levels of vitamin C inactivated poliomyelitis virus and, in animal experiments, provided a small amount of protection against paralysis when these organisms were injected into the nervous system.[40] In healthy young medical students, 1 gram of vitamin C per day substantially increased blood levels of three of the body's four most important antibodies.[41] Japanese studies have reported vitamin C in high doses is effective against hepatitis, measles, mumps, viral pneumonia, herpes zoster, herpes facialis, stomatitis apthosa, and certain types of meningitis.

In one American study, one quart of orange juice (approximately 500 mg. Vitamin C) given immediately before infection protected against Rubella virus in people. Half that much orange juice consumed daily for a week was reported to give some protection against the common cold virus, too.

A Yugoslavian researcher injected lethal rabies virus into the bloodstream of guinea pigs. Half the animals then received injections of vitamin C twice daily. After a week, only thirty percent of the animals not given vitamin C were still alive. But sixty-five percent of the vitamin C-treated animals survived the infection.[42]

Australian experiments demonstrated that vitamin C not only remarkably enhanced the effect of antibiotics, but that it also enabled certain antibiotics to kill bacteria they previously could not. Many people suffering bacterial infections were helped through this effect, the researchers report.[43]

Vitamin C and Cancer

Recent work with vitamin C and cancer is more remarkable than any other research with cancer and vitamins and minerals, and even more remarkable than research on conventional cancer treatments such as surgery, radiation, and chemotherapy. Don't get the impression, however, that vitamin C's use in cancer therapy is a "fad" now riding the crest of sudden interest. Vitamin C's effect on resistance to cancer has been investigated for decades, in many cases long before the current "fads" in conventional treatment were developed. German doctors in 1938 gave 4 grams of vitamin C daily to cancer patients receiving radiation therapy, and reported some clinical benefit. In the 1950s, German doctors used vitamin C in doses ranging from .5 to 2 grams (with other vitamins) to aid in the treatment of terminal cancer patients, and reported that the tumors frequently stopped growing for long periods of time. British doctors gave intravenous vitamin C to terminal cancer patients in the early 1950s and reported "significant benefit" in a majority of them.[44]

It's not very difficult to understand how vitamin C could have a beneficial effect in cancer. As Dr. Ewan Cameron, Scottish surgeon who has done some of the most encouraging recent research on vitamin C and cancer, points out, many of the physiological symptoms of scurvy closely resemble what happens in cancer. In scurvy, the intracellular matrix deteriorates and the cells proliferate with little or no regard for structural or functional differentiation. A similar deterioration and proliferation takes place in cancer. For cancer to spread, or for scurvy to occur, the "ground substance" which separates the cells must weaken and deteriorate. The amount of collagen present in tissue often determines that tissue's resistance to cancer. Collagen fibers actually *dissolve* in the vicinity of invasive cancer cells.

Dr. Cameron says this dissolving of the cellular ground substance is carried out by an enzyme released by the cells themselves. Normal cell proliferation requires some loosening of the ground substance, too. But in scurvy and cancer and any other derangement of cell growth, excess amounts of this enzyme, *hyaluronidase*, are released. These excess amounts throw out the balance in the cells' environment and allow undifferentiated, uncontrolled cell proliferation. A natural inhibitor of hyaluronidase (physiological hyaluronidase inhibitor, or PHI) exists, and PHI levels have been found to *rise* during infections, trauma, wound healing, rheumatoid arthritis, and cancer—as if the body knows these are times when uncontrolled cell growth is a threat.

Dr. Cameron (and his associate, Linus Pauling) believes that vitamin C is essential for the production of PHI, and that all of the stresses mentioned above that result in an increase of PHI levels also increase the requirement for vitamin C. Dr. Cameron cites several studies which report that vitamin C levels *are,* in fact, lower in cancer patients—indicating increased utilization and need.[45]

Two studies with people suffering metastatic tumors in the bones tend to confirm Dr. Cameron's belief that vitamin C strengthens the body's resistance to cancer by strengthening the resistance to tumor growth. In one study, the bone cancer patients had high levels of substances called *mucoproteins,* which doctors believe were there as products of the breakdown of bone collagen as the tumor spread. Doctors noted that although every patient was receiving multivitamin supplements containing vitamin C, their blood levels were still extremely low. High doses of the vitamin not only brought their levels up, but also *reversed* the increase in blood levels of mucoproteins. In one of Dr. Cameron's own studies, the intense pain of bone cancer, thought to result from the pressure of the tumor's growth, was completely relieved when patients were given 10 grams of vitamin C a day.[46]

Vitamin C may also help increase the body's resistance to cancer by allowing the tumor to be "encapsulated" by a tough wall of collagen. Dr. Cameron and other physicians report that such a barrier often occurs in certain cancer patients. It may be part of the body's natural cancer-resistance mechanism, which becomes severely weakened when the increased requirement for vitamin C is not met.[47]

The body's immune system is also important to resisting cancer. Many researchers believe that one of the functions of the immune system is to destroy cancer cells before they become a significant danger to the body, but that this mechanism somehow goes awry when cancer begins to spread. As we've seen, vitamin C can have a powerful effect on boosting the power of the immune system. Many cancer researchers have looked at some of these effects with particular reference to how they might apply to resistance to cancer.

For example, lymphocytes are so important to the body's resistance to cancer that the degree of their "infiltration" into endangered tissue is one way doctors determine the chances of the tumor's spreading or being successfully resisted. Vitamin C, of course, is essential to the production and function of the lymphocytes, and is found in higher-than-normal concentrations in them. In a vitamin C deficiency, lymphocyte activity drops. And when vitamin C is given in extra amounts, lymphocyte activity is greatly enhanced. Japanese researchers found that a 5 gram dose will boost human lymphocyte activity beyond normal and that a 10 gram dose will boost it even higher. Since cancer patients have been found to have lower-than-normal levels of vitamin C in their lymphocytes, it would seem that the relationship is a lot more than coincidental, and that perhaps bringing those vitamin C levels up should be standard practice in cancer therapy.[48]

Phagocytosis—when leukocytes devour foreign cells—is also important to the body's resistance to cancer. Several studies have shown that vitamin C is essential for phagocytosis to occur and that extra vitamin C will boost this activity. And vitamin C can stimulate the production of interferon, which also has a role in resistance to cancer.[49]

The obvious question is whether all of these effects vitamin C has on the body's resistance do any good—whether the vitamin, in fact, can help cancer patients fight their disease and whether it can help healthy people *prevent* cancer.

The earliest reports of vitamin C having benefit for cancer patients were the German reports already described. Other early studies found that radiation therapy caused vitamin C levels to drop drastically, and that from 1 to 5 grams of the vitamin were required to restore body stores. A more recent study has shown that as little as 750 mg. of vitamin C given daily to patients undergoing radiation therapy for squamous cell carcinoma of the uterine cervix significantly enhanced the response to therapy, compared with patients who weren't given the vitamin. It appears that when the increased need for vitamin C induced by radiation therapy is fulfilled, not only is the therapeutic response improved, but the side effects of the therapy are diminished.

Other early studies reporting beneficial effects on cancer patients include one in which a number of leukemia patients responded with a normal blood "picture" after injections of only 200 mg. of vitamin C, plus one in which a remission of leukemia was brought about with a daily oral dose ranging from 35 to 44 grams. Several researchers also noted that the symptoms of advanced leukemia (hemorrhaging, inflammation of the gums, bacterial infections, adrenal failure, and general malaise) are identical with the symptoms of advanced scurvy. Further tests revealed that leukemia patients have abnormally low levels of vitamin C in their leukocytes, which are normally very high in the vitamin.[50]

Dr. Ewan Cameron's work with vitamin C and cancer patients began in 1971 at the Vale of Levan Hospital in Scotland, where Dr. Cameron is Senior Consultant Surgeon. In his first trial with vitamin C, Dr. Cameron gave 10 grams a day to fifty terminally ill cancer patients. In the judgment of Dr. Cameron and other doctors, none of them could be helped by conventional cancer treatments. Some received 10 to 45 grams a day intravenously for the first ten days. But most started out right away with their oral 10-gram dose.

Dr. Cameron, and his associate in the trial, Dr. Allan Campbell, divided the responses into six groups. Seventeen patients had no response to the therapy. Ten patients had "minimal response," meaning they had some benefit either in the relief of pain or in the slight extension of their survival. Eleven patients' tumors slowed down in their growth; these patients experienced relief from pain, clinical improvement, and substantial extension of their survival time over what was originally expected in light of their condition. Three patients' tumors stopped growing entirely. In five patients, the tumors actually shrank, resulting in considerable remission of symptoms and extension of survival time. In four patients, the tumor hemorrhaged almost immediately after beginning vitamin C therapy. These patients died soon thereafter.

Dr. Cameron and his coworkers report that the great majority of these patients obviously experienced some benefit from the vitamin C treatment. Subjectively, the patients themselves, their relatives, the nursing staff, and many other doctors noted improvement. Pain, distress, pressure effects (headache), effusions into the lungs and other body cavities, levels of blood in the urine, jaundice, and other clinical features improved, too. And biochemical measurements, such as blood levels of vitamin C, leukocyte and lymphocyte levels of vitamin C, and levels of hyaluronidase and PHI all showed that vitamin C was providing a beneficial effect.[51]

Most of the people from that first group eventually died of their cancer, although vitamin C definitely lengthened the overall survival time significantly beyond the expected point. One of the original patients is still alive, however. This man is unique because he was not "untreatable," exactly, but was placed on vitamin C because there was a delay in starting conventional treatment. He never got that conventional treatment because his reticulum cell sarcoma *completely* remitted—all signs and symptoms—within ten days after beginning to receive 10 grams of vitamin C intravenously per day. So complete was his recovery that the doctors considered that they had made a mistake in the original diagnosis. (But all consultant physicians, surgeons, pathologists, radiologists, and radiotherapists rechecked the tests and agreed that the man indeed did have serious malignant disease.)

Over the next few months, the man's vitamin C treatments were reduced and finally eliminated. *Within a month, he was back in the hospital with the same symptoms and signs as before.* This time, slightly more vitamin C was required to bring about a remission (20 grams intravenously for two weeks, and 12.5 grams per day orally afterwards). The remission was just as complete, but it did take longer. The man returned to work—as a long-haul truck driver—and remains fit and well with no signs of active cancer.[52]

Since that first group of patients, Dr. Cameron has treated over 500 "untreatable" cancer patients with vitamin C. He has reported two main overall effects: an increase in the average survival time in most of the patients (ninety percent) of from 2.7 to 4.2 times the expected and measured time in comparable cases, and a quite remarkable extension of survival time in a few of them (about ten percent). Among the former group, the life extension might be a matter of days, weeks, or several months. But in the latter group, it means some of them were restored to the life expectancy they would have had if they didn't have cancer. Dr. Cameron has also reported that these patients do not generally experience the typical long, slow death of cancer, but that they go about their normal lives and then suddenly take ill and die within a few days. Dr. Cameron (and Dr. Pauling) is convinced that vitamin C would have even greater benefit if it were used in the treatment of cancer in the earlier stages, before the patient has already been pronounced terminal.[53]

Japanese doctors have recently confirmed the beneficial effect of vitamin C in cancer by treating a series of terminal patients with 5 grams or more per day, and using conventional treatments plus little or no vitamin C (average 1.5 grams per day). The average survival time of the patients who got little or no vitamin C was 43 days, while that of the vitamin C treated patients was 201 days—and that figure was still growing at the time of the report, because six of the people were still alive. Vitamin C-treated patients also experienced the same improvement in well-being, appetite, alertness, and desire to return to ordinary life noted by Dr. Cameron's patients.[54]

Will vitamin C *prevent* cancer? Several studies have established a definite relationship between vitamin C intake and incidence of cancer. Numerous researchers report that people with gastric cancer tend to have diets lower in vitamin C, and lower in foods containing vitamin C such as fresh fruits and vegetables. Many researchers attribute the decline in gastric cancer in the United States to the overall increased intake of vitamin C. Doctors at Tulane University have developed and tested the concept that supplemental doses of vitamin C can prevent malignant degeneration of bladder cancer.[55]

Several researchers have reported that vitamin C can help

keep rectal polyps from developing into malignant tumors. People with *familial polyposis* are generally at high risk for development of malignant cancer of the rectum. Surgical removal of the polyps usually gives only temporary relief, since the polyps recur soon thereafter. Treatment with vitamin C, however (one gram, three times a day, in a time-release capsule), resulted in regression of the polyps in five out of eight people. The doctors believe that vitamin C neutralizes carcinogenic chemicals in the colon, which are formed by bacteria working on the contents of the intestine.[56] Increasing vitamin C intake, eating more bran, and lowering fat in the diet also resulted in a decrease in the amount of potentially carcinogenic material in the colon, in a study involving people not necessarily suffering from polyposis.[57]

Other studies have demonstrated that vitamin C can protect hairless mice from the cancer-causing effects of ultraviolet light, and that vitamin C detoxifies carcinogenic chemicals such as nitrites and aromatic hydrocarbons.[58]

With all this evidence that vitamin C does considerable good in the fight against cancer, you might think vitamin C would be on the mind, if not the shelf, of every doctor who treats cancer patients. Sadly, it is not. For many reasons, some of which are economic, some of which are merely attributable to the intransigence and arrogance of the medical profession, there seems to be great resistance to acknowledging vitamin C's potential contribution to cancer therapy and prevention. Linus Pauling, who all agree is the "champion" of vitamin C's use in cancer and other diseases, has had a hard time getting the National Cancer Institute to grant funds to carry on more research on vitamin C and cancer. Such a situation is difficult enough to understand. But it becomes even more so when you realize that over the past twenty-five years, drug therapy for cancer has *grown* in popularity, even though it has brought about no improvement in survival rates for most human cancers![59]

Neither Dr. Cameron nor Dr. Pauling claims vitamin C is a cure for cancer. What they and other researchers are *demon-*

strating, however, is that vitamin C plays a vital role in treating cancer *and preventing it in healthy people*. They are proving that cancer patients definitely need a lot more vitamin C than they are presently getting in their diet. And they are making it more and more plain that perhaps the rest of us should get more than we're getting, too, whether by increasing vitamin C-rich foods in our diet or by taking supplements. Dr. Cameron, by the way, takes 4 grams of vitamin C supplements each day. He says he's saving the higher doses for when he needs them—if he ever does.

Vitamin C and Bone Disease

Paget's Disease is a noncancerous metabolic bone disease in which the bones become inflamed, deformed, and very painful. Because of reports that vitamin C had helped people with disc lesions, bone tumors, and other bone diseases, British doctors decided to test whether vitamin C could help people with Paget's disease. Drugs usually given for the relief of pain in this disease are extremely expensive. A group of sixteen people with the disease were given 3 grams of vitamin C daily for two weeks. Three received complete relief from pain, five reported partial relief. One patient who was relieved of pain had been suffering for fifteen years with no relief. The doctors concluded that since vitamin C is inexpensive, safe, and easy to administer, it is the preferred first treatment for Paget's disease before expensive drug therapy is begun.[60]

Vitamin C and Arthritis

Several studies have demonstrated a potential place for vitamin C in the treatment of arthritis. One such study found that low vitamin C levels in the tissues increase the chances for and intensity of the allergic response, and that increased concentration of vitamin C could act as an anti-inflammatory agent.[61] Another study found that a combination of vitamin C, bioflavonoids, and enzymes was more effective in reducing inflammation than seven nonsteroid anti-inflammatory drugs.[62] And a Canadian study found that high concentrations of vitamin C (in test tube cultures) were more effective than aspirin in reducing the growth of arthritic cells. Vitamin C *completely destroyed* the arthritic cells, whereas aspirin merely inhibited their growth.[63]

Vitamin C and Mental Health

Orthomolecular psychiatrists and physicians often make use of high doses of vitamin C in the treatment of schizophrenia and other forms of mental illness. Schizophrenic patients are reported to have lower concentrations of vitamin C in their blood than normal people, even when dietary intakes are equal. A study of forty male patients, thirty-four with schizophrenia, four with manic-depressive psychosis, and two with general dementia, tested vitamin C's effectiveness at relatively low doses. Half the men were given 1 gram a day for three weeks. The other half received a placebo. They were then tested on standard mental health scales, which revealed that there was significant improvement in their depression, mania, paranoia, and overall personality functioning.

Another study found that 81 out of 106 patients hospitalized for schizophrenia had deficiencies of vitamin C.[64] A Canadian study revealed that high intake of vitamin C could increase the production of a natural body substance (cAMP) which is known for its role in many vital processes, including the availability of neurotransmitter chemicals necessary for proper nervous function. (cAMP concentrations are also associated with cell growth, the immune response, and control of blood sugar. Vitamin C's ability to stimulate cAMP production and activity could help explain its role in resistance to cancer and infections, and its ability to lower insulin requirements in diabetics.)[65]

A British study of the effects of low doses of vitamin supplements (100 mg. of vitamin C) found a relationship between high concentrations of vitamin C and increased friendliness and warmth, better concentration, and improved sleep patterns.[66]

A Czechoslovakian study found that vitamin C supplements (1 gram per day) improved the "vigilance" of a group of coal miners, resulting in fewer accidents and injuries on the job.[67] In an American study, children from matched pairs of twins given from 500 to 1000 mg. of vitamin C a day for five months not only demonstrated greater resistance to colds, but also increased growth and mental alertness (measured by decreased muscle tremors), depending on age and sex.[68]

Finally, another study involving those dentists and their wives who were surveyed about their intake of vitamins and their health revealed that those who consumed more than 400 mg. of vitamin C each day had about half as much *fatigue* as the people who got less than 100 mg. per day in their diet.[69]

The overall implication of these studies is that vitamin C levels in the diet can have an effect on mental functioning. Considering all the factors (stresses) that can increase the need for vitamin C, it's reasonable to assume that our mental health can be affected in small ways if vitamin C levels fall too far.

Severely mentally ill people are most likely not suffering from a normal deficiency, however. Their increased needs stem from metabolic defects which only high doses of the vitamin can correct. Keep in mind that vitamin C concentrations are but one of the many factors that affect the nervous system.

Vitamin C and Detoxification

Vitamin C helps protect the body from the effects of several common poisons and pollutants. In one study, vitamin C (in doses equivalent to several grams for a human) *completely* protected animals from the effects of lethal doses of alcohol. All of the vitamin C-treated animals survived the lethal dose, but only thirty percent of the other animals did. The researchers concluded that vitamin C accelerated the clearance of alcohol from the bloodstream.[70]

Vitamin C also helps protect us from cadmium, an industrial pollutant which has found its way into our air, water, food, and just about everything else. Cadmium is not only impossible to avoid, but insidious in its effects: kidney damage with resultant high blood pressure, anemia, and gastrointestinal dysfunction resulting in malabsorption of nutrients. Several studies have shown that low levels of vitamin C in the diet and body tissues correspond to high susceptibility to cadmium toxicity. In quail fed toxic amounts of cadmium, vitamin C supplementation completely prevented the toxic effects of the poison.[71] In experiments with rats, feeding them vitamin C and iron supplements not only prevented the toxic effects of cadmium, but also reversed toxicity in animals already experiencing them.[72]

Vitamin C also helps protect the body against lead poisoning. Vitamin C supplements (with zinc) dropped the blood levels of lead in workers at a storage battery factory—*while the men were still on the job and exposed to lead every day.*[73] Several studies have shown that vitamin C also protects against the toxic effects of nitrates in processed food (they produce a blood disorder called methemoglobinemia),[74] vanadium (an industrial pollutant),[75] PCBs (polychlorinatedbiphenyl),[76] and organophosphate insecticides (parathion and malathion).[77]

Vitamin C protects us against some of the toxic effects of steroid drugs, which include depressed immunity to infections, and slow wound healing.[78] Paracetamol (commonly known as acetaminophen) can cause liver dysfunction and damage. However, 500 mg. of vitamin C, three times a day, protected even undernourished male volunteers given high doses of paracetamol from this effect. Vitamin C protected mice from lethal doses of the drug in another experiment by the same researchers.[79] Since many people take this drug for chronic conditions, it would seem to be a good idea if vitamin C were included in the tablet formulation.

Nitrosamines are carcinogenic substances formed from nitrates and nitrites in foods. These chemicals are added as preservatives in many processed foods, especially smoked meats. Vitamin C prevents the formation of nitrosamines when it is present in the stomach at the same time as the nitrites or nitrates.[80]

Finally, one handy use of vitamin C is to dechlorinate water. A pinch of powdered vitamin C added to a gallon of water will instantaneously neutralize the chlorine. The taste and odor of the chlorine will also disappear.

Vitamin C and Absorption of Other Nutrients

Vitamin C taken with iron (contained in food or in a supplement) increases the absorption of the mineral by as much as a thousand percent, depending on the amount of vitamin C taken and the content of the food. The researchers who carried out this experiment concluded that a 300 mg. supplement of vitamin C taken only at breakfast would increase iron absorption over the day by a factor of two, but that dividing the dose over the day would increase absorption by a factor of three.[81]

Vitamin C also enhances absorption of calcium[82] and certain essential amino acids (components of protein).[83]

Vitamin C inhibits the destruction of thiamine by tannin, if present at the beginning of the reaction. And it *reverses* the reaction if added to the contents of the gut within a half hour.[84]

Chromium in its trivalent molecular form is an essential nutrient. But in its hexavalent form, it's toxic. Vitamin C converts hexavalent chromium to trivalent chromium.[85]

HOW MUCH VITAMIN C DO WE NEED?

The RDA for vitamin C ranges from 35 mg. for infants to 60 mg. for adults, 80 mg. for pregnant women, and 100 mg. for lactating women. These amounts seem puny compared to the doses of the vitamin used in experiments and studies described in this chapter. Is it possible that so small an

amount can fulfill the requirement for all the functions
vitamin C apparently has? How much vitamin C is enough?

First, it's important to understand that the RDA for vitamin
C is supposed to be the amount that will prevent the development of scurvy in normal people. By "scurvy," the scientists
who set the standard mean the acute form. But many doctors
and researchers feel that scurvy can occur with a more insidious development of symptoms, or that *localized scurvy* can
occur in certain areas or tissues of the body, resulting in a
whole range of possible disorders. There is enough evidence to
convince several scientists and doctors that "chronic, latent
scurvy is prevalent" in modern society.[86] This means that vast
numbers of people are not getting enough vitamin C to help
build their resistance to diseases either as minor as bleeding
gums and easy bruising, or as devastating as cancer and heart
disease.

Many factors can contribute to a vitamin C deficiency or an
increased need for the vitamin. For example, vitamin C
deficiencies have been found in people who don't like "acid"
foods.[87] Smokers, as a rule, have lower tissue levels of vitamin
C than nonsmokers. Smoking is known to directly deplete the
vitamin C levels.[88] This depletion could be one factor in
smokers' higher death rate from cancer and heart disease.

Studies of hospital patients have found many of them with
low blood levels of vitamin C, resulting from either the stress
of treatment or disease or the inadequacy of hospital nutrition.[89] A check of vitamin C content in a home for the elderly
found there wasn't enough to meet even the RDA.[90]

Infants fed on cow's milk, without supplementation with
vitamin C or fresh orange juice, make up the largest single
group of humans with clinically recognized scurvy in the
United States and Canada. Breastfed infants, on the other
hand, have an extremely low rate of scurvy.[91] Vitamin C levels
are lower than normal in people with liver disease, a deficiency which can result in an increase in the toxicity of drugs
used to treat the diseases.[92] Hyperthyroid patients also tend to
have lower than normal tissue levels of vitamin C.[93]

Several drugs can cause a vitamin C deficiency. Among them are: adrenal corticosteroids (which can actually induce scurvy symptoms); estrogen-containing drugs such as oral contraceptives and menopausal drugs; barbiturates; and tetracycline. Aspirin can increase urinary excretion of vitamin C by a factor of three.[94]

Any condition which results in an increase in blood levels of copper can also increase the need for vitamin C.[95] Many people are not aware that considerable copper can enter the body through water which is piped through copper plumbing. Apparently, vitamin C is involved in the detoxification of excess levels of copper.

All of these facts don't really answer the question of how much vitamin C we need in our diet or through supplementation. And it doesn't make answering it any easier—although it may reduce your anxiety—to realize that *the experts can't agree, either.* Not even the scientists who agree that we need more than the RDA of vitamin C, nor those who agree that we need more than our food can practically provide, agree on just how much we should take.

One argument is that animals who synthesize their own vitamin C will make *more* of the vitamin when they are stressed. For example, when a rat is stressed, its vitamin C production triples. A human would have to take from 5 to 15 grams to equal such a boost in vitamin C available to the tissues.[96]

Dr. Roger Williams answers the question by saying that it depends on how much we consider we "need" and how much we consider "a luxury." Dr. Williams says one level of intake will prevent acute scurvy, and that condition might be considered "health" by some people; whereas many people aren't satisfied with that, and want "better" health, or "optimal" health. One of the things these people who want optimal health will do is get more vitamin C. Furthermore, because of wide variations in requirements among individuals, what helps create optimum health for one person may not be enough for another.[97]

Would Nature leave us in such a situation? Is it "natural" to need 500 or 1000 or 10,000 mg. of vitamin C in order to be healthy? Remember, the RDA is not based on natural facts or observations, but on arbitrary decisions by a committee. In the same way, Nature's requirements are not based on observations of what's "fair," or politically or economically easy. Primitive people, who might be considered closer to Nature, ate a diet that was much higher in vitamin C than the modern diet. They ate their fruits and vegetables fresh and raw. When they ate meat, they ate the organs that were highest in vitamin C first and left the muscle meats for last. Many nutritional scientists and archaeologists believe that the reason people have a preference for sweet-tasting food is that in Nature sweet-tasting foods (fruits, particularly) are rich in vitamin C.

Many researchers cite the amount of vitamin C necessary to maintain tissue saturation as the optimally required dose. Under normal, unstressed circumstances, 120 mg. usually suffices. But this requirement rises considerably during any kind of stress.[98] Furthermore, this may not take into account that *local tissue deficiencies of vitamin C may require many times more vitamin C than it takes to saturate other parts of the body*. Remember, in many of the experimental therapeutic uses of vitamin C, the affected tissues were often deficient in vitamin C even when blood and other tissue levels were normal. In a test of the effect of vitamin C on elderly hospital patients, 1 gram was given daily to a group which was found to have blood plasma and leukocyte levels of vitamin C that "overlapped" with those seen in scurvy. The daily dose of vitamin C *did* improve their health and well-being, but their leukocyte levels of the vitamin still did not rise all the way to normal.[99]

The more research reports you read, the more it seems that the 60 mg. RDA is ridiculously low.

TOXICITY OF VITAMIN C

Vitamin C is nontoxic. Media reports of its toxicity and

speculation of its toxicity by some doctors are ungrounded in fact. Reports of its *intravenous* use in humans at doses ranging from a few grams to over 200 grams all agree that no serious side effects are produced.[100] In healthy people, vitamin C in doses of 4 grams or more per day may produce flatulence, transient colic, and diarrhea in some individuals. High doses can also slightly increase urinary oxalate excretion, which many believe is a factor in stone formation. Yet with all the people taking very high doses of vitamin C, there have been no reports of stones actually forming in anyone taking high doses of vitamin C. The supposed diuretic effects of vitamin C were not observed by Dr. Cameron and his associates.[101]

One effect of high doses of vitamin C that is still controversial is the so-called "rebound" effect, in which a person taking high doses will become deficient in the vitamin when the dosage is suddenly reduced. Some studies have shown that the body "adjusts" to very high intake of vitamin C by becoming less efficient in absorbing it and more efficient in excreting it. If this were so, suddenly dropping from a high dose to a low dose would rapidly deplete body stores. Although some studies have shown that there is no "rebound" effect and that body stores remain high long after long-term high doses (2 grams per day), *higher* doses *may* require gradual "weaning" to a lower daily dose.[102]

SOURCES OF VITAMIN C

The richest natural sources of vitamin C are citrus fruits and their juices, strawberries, cantaloupes, raw vegetables— especially peppers, parsley, broccoli, cauliflower, kale, brussels sprouts, turnip greens, cabbage, tomatoes, potatoes, and bean sprouts. Vitamin C levels in these items vary according to how they're grown, stored, and prepared. The amount of sunlight determines vitamin C content, more sunlight producing more of the vitamin. Furthermore, vitamin C is vulnerable to oxidation, so storage can expose it to considerable losses. Since the vitamin is water-soluble, steaming for prolonged periods, washing, soaking, and canning result in severe losses. Storage of citrus juice at warm temperatures results in almost total loss of vitamin C content.

Vitamin C is available in supplemental form in a wide range of doses, from a few milligrams to over 1 gram (1000 mg.). Vitamin C tablets advertised as "natural" or "rose hips" or "acerola" should be carefully examined before purchase. These forms of vitamin C are usually composed of some synthetic vitamin C with the addition of small quantities of acerola berry or rose hips. There's nothing wrong with "synthetic" vitamin C. It's produced by the fermentation of glucose, basically the same way it's produced in Nature. However, "natural" vitamin C tablets are often sold for many times the price of the same strength tablet labeled plainly "ascorbic acid." Vitamin C is also available as sodium ascorbate. Doctors who use this claim it's every bit as potent as ascorbic acid. And it is used interchangeably with ascorbic acid in many experiments and therapeutic trials. Persons wishing to keep the sodium in their diet as low as possible would be wise to avoid this form of the vitamin, however.

Vitamin C is also available in pure powdered form, which is by far the least expensive way to obtain the vitamin.

14

Vitamin D

Most people think of vitamin D as the "sunshine vitamin," which is a good way to think of it, and as the "children's vitamin," which is a bad way to think of it. Vitamin D is just as important to adults as it is to children, and for many of the same reasons.

Viltamin D is unique for two reasons: it's synthesized by the body when the skin is exposed to sufficient sunlight; and because it's involved in regulating the function of specific organs, it's also a hormone.

WHAT VITAMIN D DOES

Vitamin D's primary function is to enhance intestinal absorption of calcium and phosphorus in order to maintain adequate blood levels of the two minerals for calcification of bone and cartilage. As a hormone, vitamin D regulates the activity of an enzyme, l-ahydroxylase, which is necessary to convert vitamin D to its active form in the body. Blood levels of vitamin D and calcium determine the amount of enzyme activity. When blood levels of calcium and vitamin D drop, enzyme activity increases in order to produce more of the metabolically active vitamin. In this way, we are protected against "low spots" in our intake of calcium and vitamin D. However, if enough of the metabolically active vitamin is produced—either because of a severe deficiency in calcium or a toxic overdose of vitamin D—calcium will be mobilized from the bones, too.

Vitamin D also plays a role in the proper mineralization of bone at the site of the bone itself. Little is known about exactly how this occurs, however.

Vitamin D also appears to be important to the structure and function of the thyroid and pituitary glands, since one of the effects of a deficiency is malfunction of those organs.

Low levels of extra vitamin D in the diet have also been found to lower the blood cholesterol.[1] Even though the amount of vitamin D necessary to achieve this effect is far from toxic, not enough is known about this to recommend supplements of vitamin D for people with high cholesterol.

WHAT HAPPENS WHEN VITAMIN D DEMAND EXCEEDS SUPPLY

A deficiency in vitamin D results in severely diminished absorption of calcium and phosphorus from the intestine. Urinary and fecal levels of these minerals will rise and blood levels will drop. To maintain normal blood levels of calcium (necessary for functions other than bone mineralization—see Calcium chapter), calcium will be mobilized from the bones. In adults, this softening of the bones is called *osteomalacia*. In children, whose bones are still growing, calcium and phosphorus are not deposited in the cartilage matrix, and the cartilage is not replaced as it should be; so the bones become swelled with cartilage at the ends and soft and malformed in the middle. This is called *rickets*. Vitamin D deficiency during development can also result in thin, irregular tooth enamel.[2]

Low dietary intake and blood levels of vitamin D (and calcium) have also been associated with high blood levels of lead. The low blood and tissue levels of calcium are believed to mobilize lead from the bones and deposit it in the soft tissues of the body, where it can do more harm.[3]

Classic Symptoms of Vitamin D Deficiency

The early signs of rickets are irritability and restlessness. Because any of a hundred factors can also cause a child to be irritable and restless, the onset of rickets is considered insidious. An infant with rickets walks or crawls late (another characteristic caused by many things), and the cranial fontanelles are delayed in closing. One of the first unmistakable signs is a soft, yielding skull. The ribs will bend and the ends of the long bones will swell. Mechanical and gravitational stress will eventually cause bowed legs, knock knees, depressions in the chest, and pigeon-chest deformity of the rib cage.

In rachitic children, the teeth erupt late, decay early, and are malformed. Low blood levels of calcium may also result in neuromuscular hyperirritability, spasms of the wrist and foot, general spasticity, and convulsive seizures.

Osteomalacia

When vitamin D deficiency occurs in adults, the bones are robbed of their minerals. This demineralization is usually more severe in the spine, pelvis, and legs. The bones of the spine soften and compress, the long bones bow, and the pelvis compresses. These deformities result in pain, and the pain is aggravated by muscle strain, weight bearing, pressure, or sudden movements. Sometimes incorrect diagnoses of muscular rheumatism, arthritis, or herniated disc will be made. Narrowing of the birth canal, scoliosis, and shortening of the spine can also occur. Muscle weakness in the lower limbs may lead to a waddling gait.

Osteomalacia can also result in blood levels of calcium low

enough to produce muscle cramps, burning and tingling, numbness, spasms, or convulsions.

Treatment for osteomalacia can require doses of vitamin D from 2000 international units (IU) up to 40,000 IU.

Osteoporosis

Osteomalacia and osteoporosis are often confused. Osteoporosis also involves demineralization of the bones, but rather than softening, the bones become porous and brittle. Osteoporosis is usually associated with old age, with menopausal changes in hormone balance, and with skeletal disuse caused by lack of exercise. Recent research indicates, however, that dietary calcium and vitamin D are also important factors.

Osteoporosis can be a very dangerous condition. Because the bones grow weaker, they sometimes fracture from the very stress of gravity. Any kind of actual trauma can be a catastrophe for someone with osteoporotic bones. Falls are among the leading causes of accidental death, and fractures account for about three-fourths of the deaths from falls. Elderly people and females are particularly at risk. Osteoporosis is definitely an important factor, because a substantial percentage of these lethal fractures involve no discernible trauma. The bones just give way spontaneously.

Adequate vitamin D (and calcium) can prevent osteoporosis. A study at the Mayo Clinic found that vitamin D and calcium (2 to 2.5 grams) supplements could slow and in some cases actually stop the turnover of bone in osteoporotic people. The amount of vitamin D used in the supplements was 50,000 IU per day for a year. No side effects were reported, and none of the people taking supplements suffered further vertebral fractures during the treatment.[4]

Loss of bone from the alveolar ridge of the jaw (the sockets in which the teeth are embedded) can result in lost teeth *and* lost dentures. In light of several studies that reported increased bone density in osteoporotic people given calcium and vitamin D supplements, a group of dental researchers tested the effect of 750 mg. of calcium and 375 units of vitamin D per day on alveolar bone demineralization. These supplementary amounts were substantially less than amounts used in most studies of this type. Nonetheless, the people who received the supplements experienced from thirty-four to thirty-nine percent *less bone loss*. This experiment suggests that merely making sure that *adequate* levels of calcium and vitamin D are in the diet can significantly inhibit osteoporosis.[5]

A British study revealed a definite association between spontaneous fractures in the long bones of people suffering rheumatoid arthritis and a deficiency of vitamin D. The people were found to have diets adequate in protein, calories, and calcium. However, they were very low in vitamin D. In many of these cases, a vicious cycle starts when aging people stay at home and neglect to go out in the sunshine and exercise. Their lack of activity weakens their appetite, provides less good food, and keeps them out of the sunshine where they might get enough vitamin D to keep their bones healthy. But as they get more housebound, they get weaker and their bone health suffers further.[6]

Bone demineralization usually begins between the ages of thirty and forty, so the above information is not of interest only to the elderly. As a matter of fact, doctors have suggested that dietary changes made *before* demineralization starts will help prevent the process from ever occurring. Many doctors insist that osteoporosis begins when hormone levels change during menopause. But recent research reveals that the loss of bone begins *before* estrogen levels drop. Jaw demineralization may be the first sign. Raising the dietary intake of calcium and vitamin D appears to be the best preventive measure.[7]

Vitamin D and Kidney Disease

Many of the symptoms of renal failure are similar to those of vitamin D deficiency. Since the kidneys are essential to the metabolism of vitamin D, researchers have suspected that some of these symptoms actually do result from a metabolic deficiency of the active form of the vitamin. Tests have born this out, since long term treatment with metabolically active vitamin D has successfully treated both the osteitis (bone inflammation) and osteomalacia associated with renal disease. These symptoms had not responded to normal therapeutic dosages of vitamin D. Doses as high as 200,000 units per day had previously been required.[8]

HOW MUCH VITAMIN D DO WE NEED?

The RDA for vitamin D is 400 units per day for infants, children, adolescents, pregnant women, and lactating mothers. The RDA for all other adults declines with age from 400 to 300 units from ages nineteen to twenty-two, and to 200 units beyond age twenty-three. This fact is additional evidence of how useless the RDA is as a guideline for nutritional adequacy. It totally ignores the evidence that adults and the elderly need vitamin D to prevent osteoporosis and osteomalacia.

Vitamin D deficiency is more common than it should be. Many factors can contribute to a vitamin D deficiency, including diet, intestinal malabsorption, gastric surgery, and insufficient exposure to sunlight. Two California doctors were surprised to find deficient blood levels of vitamin D in thirty-two percent of their patients.[9] A British Government committee estimated the prevalence of malnutrition including vitamin D deficiency to be about three percent of the nation's elderly.[10] And osteoporosis affects more than 14 million women in the United States.[11] A Boston study found that vitamin D, calcium, and phosphorus intakes were lower than normal, and lower than other vegetarians, in children of macrobiotic vegetarians. None of the symptoms of rickets was found, however.[12]

Several drugs can interfere with the metabolism of vitamin D and cause a deficiency, including liquid paraffin taken as a laxative, anticonvulsant drugs (phenturide, primidone, phenytoin, phenobarbitone), the hypnotic glutethimide, and corticosteroids such as prednisone.[13]

TOXICITY OF VITAMIN D

Vitamin D is fat-soluble and stored in the liver. Excessive doses of vitamin D mobilize calcium and phosphorus from the bones and redeposit them in the soft tissues such as the blood vessels, kidneys, lungs, and heart. Preliminary symptoms of toxicity include loss of appetite, thirst, urgency of urination, vomiting, headache, and diarrhea. There is a wide range of susceptibility among adults. Some adults have shown signs of toxicity with as little as 50,000 units per day for a few weeks, whereas others tolerate ten times that much for a year. Calcification of the kidneys occurs when doses reach 300,000 to 500,000 units a day over a long period of time.[14] No toxicity from vitamin D synthesis stimulated by the sun has even been reported. Apparently, the body regulates the amounts that are synthesized, stored, and used.

Since calcification is one of the effects of toxic doses of vitamin D, some have proposed a role for vitamin D in the development of arteriosclerosis. A study, however, of blood levels of vitamin D among heart patients found that their levels were no higher than those of healthy people.[15]

SOURCES OF VITAMIN D

Natural sources of vitamin D are scarce, unless you include sunshine. Fish, especially fish with heavy amounts of oil in the flesh (saltwater fish, salmon, sardines, herring) are good sources. Liver, egg yolk, and summer milk are also good sources. Most current dietary sources of vitamin D are actually foods which have been "fortified" with synthetic vitamin D.

Vitamin D supplements are available in doses ranging from a few units to several hundred units. Two forms of the vitamin are used, vitamin D_2 and D_3. D_2 is the synthetic form, and is also called calciferol, or activated ergosterol. D_3 is the "naturally occurring" form and is usually obtained from fish liver oils.

Vitamin D is, of course, the sunshine vitamin. When the skin is exposed to ultraviolet light at the correct wavelength, vitamin D is synthesized below the surface. There is some question among scientists as to which is more important as a source of vitamin D, sunlight or diet. A day in the sun in northern parts of America during the months of March through October can provide as much as 10,000 units of vitamin D. During the winter months, however, very little is provided.[16]

In the previously mentioned study of blood levels of lead in children, blood levels of vitamin D were found to reflect dietary intake regardless of the season of the year. However, the children were all dark-skinned and none spent more than three hours a day out-of-doors.[17] A British study found that children's blood concentrations of vitamin D were higher in August than in February, and that children who had a vacation at the seashore the previous summer had higher levels than children who didn't. There was no correlation between dietary intake of vitamin D and blood levels. Among adults, the researchers found that blood levels of D^3 were higher than blood levels of D^2 (obtained from a fortified diet), even after supplementation with D^2. The researchers concluded that exposure to the summer sun was a more crucial factor in blood levels of vitamin D than diet.[18]

These studies seem to suggest that the most important source of vitamin D is, indeed, the sun. However, we should not adopt the attitude that supplementation is worthless. All of the therapeutic studies used vitamin D supplements to raise blood levels. People who *cannot* get enough exposure to the sun, as well as people who have some of the conditions which may cause a deficiency (mentioned above) should no doubt use supplements. When buying supplements of vitamin D, always prefer D^3 from fish liver oil, and always stay away from enteric-coated or time release capsules, since these may be inadequately absorbed. Some doctors warn against buying vitamin D in multivitamin supplements where its proximity to other substances may enhance destruction by oxidation.[19]

15

Vitamin E

Vitamin E's reputation as the "sex vitamin" is an example of good publicity for the wrong reason. Vitamin E *does* have a role in the health of the reproductive system, a role which may extend into our everyday sex lives. But the most exciting things about vitamin E have really very little to do with directly influencing sex.

Vitamin E earned its reputation quite early. The very first published report of research establishing its essentiality, by doctors Herbert Evans and Katherine Bishop, did so on the basis of its role in the reproductive system. Rats were maintained on a diet free of vitamin E, but unlike most other deficiency syndromes, no physical symptoms appeared: "The animals are of splendid size, sleek coated and active." They grew normally and had every "appearance of health." Except, as the researchers wrote, "Practically all of such animals are sterile."

They subsequently found that a substance in fresh raw

lettuce leaves, whole wheat, oats, wheat germ, and meat prevented the fetal rebsorption that was keeping the rats from bearing young. Borrowing "tocos" and "phero," Greek words meaning "childbirth" and "to bring forth," they named the substance *tocopherol*. Thus the "sex vitamin" was born.[1]

WHAT VITAMIN E DOES

Vitamin E's primary role appears to be as an antioxidant. In this role, vitamin E protects fatty acids (oils) against oxidation and rancidity. This role grows in importance when you realize that all the cells and subcellular membranes of the body contain a sizeable portion of fatty acids which require such protection against oxidation. These fatty acids (usually polyunsaturated) serve vital roles in the cells, and scientists believe oxidation of them causes not only many diseases but some of the symptoms of aging as well.

Many enzyme systems are impaired during a vitamin E deficiency. However, no exact function for vitamin E in a particular enzyme reaction has been found. Some scientists believe the effect on enzyme systems may be due to oxidation (or peroxidation) of the tissue components of the enzyme system.

Vitamin E's protective effects on the cell have been demonstrated in several studies with red blood cells. One study involved a group of people given 600 IU of vitamin E per day for ten days, then tested for the ability of their red blood cells to resist oxidative "aging" when exposed to light and excess oxygen. Whereas red blood cells from nonsupplemented people were completely "budded" (this refers to oxidative damage), those from the supplemented group were only about eight percent budded.[2]

As red blood cells age, they become less "filterable." One study with rats found that vitamin E-supplemented animals had red blood cells which were remarkably resistant to the aging effect of lead poisoning. Red blood cells from E-supplemented rats which were also poisoned with lead were still more filterable than red blood cells from animals fed no lead but who received a diet deficient in vitamin E. Normal aging of the red blood cells from the supplemented animals also failed to produce any significant difference in their filterability.[3]

A study of cystic fibrosis patients with vitamin E deficiencies found that their red blood cells had greatly increased susceptibility to abnormal oxidative destruction. Although they all had biochemical signs of increased destruction of red blood cells, none yet had the symptoms of anemia. Supplements of from 100 to 200 IU of vitamin E quickly increased the survival time of their red blood cells to normal. The researchers concluded that vitamin E was essential for the maintenance of normal red blood cell structure and function.[4]

DOES VITAMIN E PROTECT US AGAINST AGING?

These and other studies have given rise to the speculation that vitamin E is the "anti-aging" vitamin, that supplements of the vitamin can protect the cells of the body against the ravages of getting older. In part, of course, this is true. One theory of aging is that substances called "free radicals" encourage oxidation of the cells and cell membranes, and that their effect snowballs as we get older. Some early studies did find that vitamin E could prolong the life of human cells grown in culture. However, subsequent experiments by the same investigators failed to duplicate the original results.[5]

Nevertheless, it's not unreasonable to grant vitamin E *some* role in resisting some of the effects of aging. Human studies have shown that in a partial vitamin E deficiency, red blood cells are destroyed about eight to ten percent faster than in an adequate vitamin E state. Researchers know two things which may lead to an expanded role for vitamin E in resisting aging. They know that there are other cells in the body with an even more rapid turnover rate than red blood cells. These cells might be even more vulnerable to low levels of vitamin E. And they know that an antioxidant's function is often directly proportional to the *amount* of the antioxidant present.[6]

There is too much evidence that oxidative damage is

involved not only in aging but in many disease states to say that vitamin E is "useless" as a protective substance. Of course, there are also too many other factors involved to believe that merely taking vitamin E supplements will protect us against aging and disease.

Vitamin E also appears to have an "oxygen sparing" effect, meaning it helps organisms get by with less oxygen than is normally required. This may be a result of promoting more efficient use of oxygen, or of merely preventing excess unrequired oxidation. In many experiments, vitamin E supplements significantly increased survival, compared to unsupplemented controls, when animals were placed in chambers with less-than-normal concentrations of oxygen. Several of the therapeutic uses of vitamin E appear to rely on this effect.[7]

Even though vitamin E has not been clearly shown to be required in any enzyme reactions involved in supplying energy to the cell, it still has an indirect connection. The integrity of the cell structure and the cell membrane are crucial to the efficient use of energy. Nutrients must pass through the cell membrane in order to reach the cell. Since vitamin E helps protect the cell from excess oxidation and promotes more efficient use of oxygen, the energy functions of the cell still depend on adequate quantities of the vitamin being present.[8]

Recent research has demonstrated that vitamin E may play a role in the synthesis and function of *prostaglandins*, hormones which regulate many organ systems, including the muscles.

WHAT HAPPENS WHEN VITAMIN E DEMAND EXCEEDS SUPPLY

In rats, vitamin E deficiency produces degeneration of the gonads, leading to loss of sperm motility in males and fetal death and resorption in the females. With this degeneration of the sex glands also comes an impairment of their function, the secretion of sex hormones. Vitamin E deficiency during development can result in a delay of puberty.[9]

Deficiency of vitamin E can also result in diminished

function of the pituitary-thyroid system. A hyperthyroid state tends to increase vitamin E requirements, since more fatty acids are concentrated in the muscles, particularly the heart muscle, and any increase in fatty acids requires more vitamin E to protect against oxidation.[10]

Degeneration and dystrophy of the skeletal, striated, and cardiac muscles also occur in a vitamin E deficiency. Degeneration of the endocrine glands, peripheral vascular system,[11] and nervous system have also been reported. In some animals, nervous system lesions take the form of softening of the brain.

The only widely recognized effect of a deficiency of vitamin E in humans is the decreased survival time of red blood cells. This was demonstrated, however, with only a partial deficiency. The subjects still received 5 IU of vitamin E per day. Also, there was not rigorous biochemical testing of the effects on other cell systems, some of which may have been more severely affected. Degeneration of the brain and spinal cord have also been reported in vitamin E-deficient children.[12]

There are no recognized basic symptoms of a vitamin E deficiency, although there are many connections between vitamin E and health problems we encounter every day. "Establishment" nutrition scientists require frank, acute deficiency symptoms, such as those which occur in scurvy, before attributing a specific disease state to a vitamin deficiency. It also seems to help if the disease occurred mainly in the *past*, or in animals. They seem reluctant to acknowledge that a vitamin, such as vitamin E or C, could have an important role in any disease that's affecting large numbers of people *today*. This is true even when there is a scientific connection between some of the physiological effects of the vitamin and the disease, as there is in vitamin C and cancer. Many of these connections occur with vitamin E.

DOES VITAMIN E ENHANCE SEX?

No known research or medical report has addressed itself to whether vitamin E has any effect on human sexual potency or libido. It is not unreasonable to assume that since vitamin E is required for the proper function of the sex glands, a deficiency will adversely affect a person's sex life. Still, sex involves more than just the sex organs and glands, more than just libido and potency. Libido and potency are usually the least of most people's problems with their sex lives.

Though vitamin E deficiency is more widespread than commonly accepted, and though such a deficiency could conceivably affect a person's sex life, no one should take extra vitamin E with the intention of taking care of all sexual problems. *All* of the vitamins, together and individually, are essential to the structure and function of many systems besides the reproductive system: the cardiovascular system, the nervous system, the endocrine system, the skeletal system, the immune system, etc. When you ask how important a vitamin is to a person's sex life, it generally depends on how important your heart, lungs, muscles, bones, skin, nerves, senses, and glands *are* to your sex life.

Vitamin E and Stress

The protective effect of vitamin E during stress was tested by feeding carbohydrates and vitamin E to rats before placing them in cold water. Rats which were deficient or "adequate" in vitamin E did not survive as long and developed more stress ulcers than the animals which got extra vitamin E and carbohydrates.[13] In humans, two weeks of supplementation with 1200 IU of vitamin E per day did not result in increased lung function during exercise. But researchers did find that *pentane*, a product of lipid peroxidation, increased during exercise and that the vitamin E supplements significantly lowered pentane production. This means that vitamin E protects against some of the damaging stress of oxidation during exercise.[14] This may help explain why vitamin E has been reported to help alleviate muscle cramps.[15]

Vitamin E and the Immune System

One of vitamin E's protective effects against aging may be

its effect on the immune system, which weakens with age. Some researchers believe free radical oxidation reactions may contribute to this decline in the immune system. A trial in which vitamin E supplements were given to mice demonstrated that the vitamin could indeed inhibit this decline. Not only was the immune response maintained throughout the lifespan of the mice, but in many cases vitamin E boosted it even higher than it had been in younger, unsupplemented mice.[16]

Vitamin E and Healing

There is a lot of "hearsay" type evidence that vitamin E is helpful in the healing of wounds, burns, and sores when applied directly to the wound. Many doctors and nutritionists recommend this treatment, though few of them report it in medical or scientific journals. The only published report was made by a dentist who uses vitamin E on viral sores in the mouths of his patients. Vitamin E is applied directly to the sores for fifteen minutes (on a gauze strip) about three times a day. He reports that success is nearly a hundred percent.[17]

Vitamin E and Heart Disease

By far the most controversial use of vitamin E is in the treatment of heart disease. This is not to say that there is less evidence of vitamin E's benefit in heart disease than in other problems, such as aging and sexual potency. But those applications of the vitamin are highly speculative, while several physicians have been using vitamin E in cardiovascular disease for more than thirty years. And since modern medicine has a substantial investment in drugs and surgery for heart disease, *any* alternative treatment is liable to attract quite a bit of resistance and controversy.

Canadian doctors Evan and Wilfrid Shute, and several of their colleagues, have been using vitamin E for more than thirty years in the treatment of various cardiovascular disorders, including thrombophlebitis, indolent ulcers of the leg, early gangrene of the extremities, thromboanginitis, coronary heart disease, angina, and rheumatic fever. They have used doses ranging from less than 100 IU to over 2400 IU on over 30,000 patients with these diseases, and they claim success in reducing symptoms, restoring function, preventing further disability, and saving lives. They also believe that vitamin E can help prevent cardiovascular disease in healthy people.[18]

With such a record behind the vitamin, it's not reasonable to say that vitamin E is of little value in the treatment of cardiovascular disease. Obviously, the Shute brothers and their colleagues haven't been deluding themselves or their patients for all these years. This doesn't imply that vitamin E is a cure for heart disease, nor would the doctors who use vitamin E advise their patients to rely on vitamin E alone to prevent the disease.

Nevertheless, there is some evidence that vitamin E may be of help. Several early studies found that a vitamin E deficiency produces severe lesions in the heart and blood vessels in animals, including cardiac insufficiency, enlargement, atrophy, heart failure, scarring of the heart and blood vessels, heart attack, and fatty deposits. Furthermore, an experiment in which supplemental vitamin E was given to animals with surgically induced heart attacks (infarctions) found that the vitamin E had increased the blood flow through the old coronary capillaries and stimulated the production of new circulatory channels to feed the heart. Infarcted hearts also were less fibrous.[19]

Vitamin E has the ability to decrease the tendency of the blood to clot. Blood platelets must "aggregate" and stick together before clotting can occur. Vitamin E appears to decrease the ability of the platelets to adhere to each other.[20] This effect is relevant to cardiovascular disease because blood clots in the wrong places and at the wrong times are a major factor. For example, in coronary arteries already narrowed by fatty deposits, a blood clot can cut off the blood supply to the heart and cause a heart attack. The same can happen in the arteries feeding the brain, causing a stroke. Sometimes, a blood clot will form in a wide artery, dislodge, and travel through the body until it lodges in a narrow vessel (embolism).

Apparently, other doctors besides the Shutes and their colleagues have taken advantage of vitamin E's ability to decrease blood clotting in cardiovascular disease. In a paper published in 1950, a group of doctors in New Orleans reports the *routine* use of 200 IU of vitamin E every eight hours for people with venous thrombosis (inflammatory blood clot in a vein). One of the authors of the report is Michael E. DeBakey, M.D., the famous heart surgeon.[21]

More recently, doctors have found hyperaggregability, or an increased tendency for the blood to clot, in two infant girls with vitamin E deficiencies. Supplements of vitamin E corrected the deficiencies and restored their blood's clotting tendencies to normal.[22]

One beneficial effect of vitamin E, the lowering of blood levels of cholesterol, has not been so decisively proved. Some researchers using 400 IU per day have not been able to lower cholesterol. Some have noticed a slight increase in HDL cholesterol, which is a good sign because HDL cholesterol is on its way out of the body. And others have managed to lower blood cholesterol with doses of about 700 IU per day.[23]

Vitamin E is necessary to prevent oxidation of fatty acids, especially unsaturated fatty acids. Fatty acid concentration in the tissues actually determines how much vitamin E is required to "cover" against damaging oxidation. When animals deficient in vitamin E are fed polyunsaturated fatty acids, muscular dystrophy results. Animal studies have shown that the heart muscle is also susceptible to damage from oxidation of fatty acids when adequate vitamin E is lacking.[24] Such heart damage in the animals resulted in "heart attacks." It's not unreasonable to make a connection between this effect and human heart disease, especially with people consuming more and more polyunsaturated fats, with their doctors' blessing, in hopes of avoiding heart disease!

Vitamin E has also been shown to be an effective vasodilator.[25] Several reports have documented the vitamin's ability to restore circulation in legs afflicted with *intermittent claudication*. Blood supply to the legs is severely hampered in this condition, making walking painful or impossible. Evidence that vitamin E is effective in this condition is so voluminous and definite that it is considered standard treatment among doctors who have no prejudice against nutritional therapy.[26]

A recent United States study attempted to find out if vitamin E had any effect on *angina*. A group of forty-eight people with angina were given 1600 IU of vitamin E per day for six months. Then they were given placebo pills. At certain intervals they were tested on exercise stress performance. The vitamin E was found to have no effect on angina; however, there was a slight improvement in their exercise performance.[27]

Another physician reports, however, that 1600 IU of vitamin E had considerable beneficial effect on a group of his patients with heart disease. Many of his patients reduced or eliminated the use of nitroglycerin tablets for their angina. However, these patients were also instructed to give up smoking, walk one and a half to five miles a day, lose weight, avoid stress, and eat a low cholesterol diet. This may have had more of an effect than the vitamin E.[28]

Finally, a Japanese study also found vitamin E to have some beneficial effect in people with cerebral arteriosclerosis. Eighty-nine patients were divided into two groups; forty-four were treated with 600 IU of vitamin E, and forty-five with a placebo. After four to six weeks, they were evaluated on several items. The group which got vitamin E scored higher in "general improvement," and the scores went higher as the length of supplementation progressed. Vitamin E also resulted in improvement in such subjective symptoms as numbness of limbs, dizziness, stiff neck, heavy feeling of head, and insomnia. And although the Shute brothers report that vitamin E can raise the blood pressure, this effect was not noted in these Japanese patients, many of whom already had high blood pressure.[29]

Vitamin E and Air Pollution

Several studies demonstrate that vitamin E helps the body protect itself against air pollution. A clue that this might be so is the fact that animals exposed to air pollution (ozone) use vitamin E faster than those breathing purified air. Ozone and nitrous oxide are the two most damaging elements of air pollution. Both exert their toxic effect by oxidizing the unsaturated fats in the cells and membranes of the lungs. Since vitamin E is a powerful antioxidant, it should help prevent some of the damage to the lungs. Researchers at Duke University have performed several experiments which have demonstrated that vitamin E does protect the lungs against oxidative damage by air pollutants. For example, in one experiment, vitamin E supplements extended by almost fifty percent the survival time of mice exposed to lethal concentrations of ozone. Other experiments by the same researchers have shown that vitamin E prevents much of the actual damage to the lungs, such as the loss of unsaturated fatty acids, and edema.[30]

Other researchers have confirmed these results.[31] One fact that emerges in many of these experiments is that the normally "adequate" dietary level of vitamin E isn't enough to protect the animals against the toxic effects of air pollution. In one study, six times the "adequate" vitamin E amount totally protected the animals, whereas those fed "adequate" levels suffered lung damage.[32]

Vitamin E and Radiation

In these days of leaking nuclear power plants, radiation is one more "pollutant" we have to worry about. One of the ways radiation damages living tissue is by encouraging free radical oxidative reactions. In one study, phospholipids (fatty acid precursors) from biologic membranes were subjected to ionizing radiation. Some of the exposed fatty acids were also mixed with either vitamin E or another antioxidant. The vitamin E was a hundred times more efficient in protecting the fatty acids against oxidation.[33] In a similar study, living cells grown in a vitamin E-enriched medium were significantly less sensitive to radiation damage than normally grown cells.[34]

Vitamin E also protects living animals against radiation. In one study, injection of vitamin E into mice exposed to lethal radiation significantly reduced the lethality.[35] And a National Cancer Institute study found that vitamin E supplements increased both median and overall survival of mice exposed to lethal radiation.[36]

These results give us no cause for comfort in the face of growing danger from leaking radiation, any more than the protective effect of vitamin E against air pollution gives us any reason to relax our clean-air standards. Nevertheless, as long as these pollutants are a fact of life, it's somewhat encouraging to know we are not entirely without natural defenses.

Vitamin E and Toxic Chemicals

Vitamin E also helps protect us against some very common poisons. Paracetemol (acetaminophen) is one such chemical. When fed to rats on a vitamin E deficient diet, the drug produced liver damage. A vitamin E "adequate" diet offered some protection. But not until *supplementary* doses of vitamin E were added to the rats' diet did the protection become almost complete.[37]

Vitamin E also protects the red blood cells from the damaging effects of lead poisoning. Both vitamin E deficiency and lead poisoning decrease the filterability of red blood cells, and when both occur at once, the effect is even greater. However, red blood cells from animals given supplements of vitamin E (in excess of "adequate" levels), were hardly affected at all by lead poisoning.[38]

Adriamycin is a commonly used anticancer and antibiotic drug which has the side effect of causing deterioration of the heart muscle, leading to congestive heart failure. Tests with animals have revealed that vitamin E supplements can prevent this damage without interfering with the anticancer activity of the drug.[39]

Vitamin E supplementation also completely protected animals against the toxic effects of (methyl) mercury.[40] And supplements of the vitamin reduced the frequency of precancerous lesions and retarded their development into tumors in mice treated with carcinogenic chemicals.[41]

Vitamin E and Infants

Newborn babies generally have less than one-fifth the blood concentration of vitamin E that their mothers have,[42] and premature babies usually have still lower concentrations. One of the effects of this deficiency can be a hemolytic anemia (anemia caused by increased rate of destruction of red blood cells). In one study, supplementary injections of vitamin E of from 125 to 150 IU per kilogram of weight (spread over the course of a week) were necessary to overcome this anemia in premature infants. The anemia was made worse in the infants who received injections of iron but no vitamin E. Apparently, iron can aggravate a vitamin E deficiency's effects on the maintenance of red blood cells.[43] At least one other study has confirmed this anemia-correcting effect of supplemental vitamin E.[44]

Premature infants are usually given oxygen immediately after birth. This therapy can have two serious side effects: bronchopulmonary dysplasia and retrolental fibroplasia. In BPD, the damage to the lung—which is actually oxidized—can lead to progressive fibrosis of the lung, lung failure, and heart failure. Respiratory distress syndrome is the nation's leading cause of infant mortality, and BPD accounts for around 5000 deaths each year. Babies born to diabetic mothers, or by Caesarean section, are also at increased risk for BPD.[45]

BPD may become much less of a threat, however, since researchers have discovered that vitamin E injections at birth can protect the infants' lung tissue from damaging oxidation. Early trials with vitamin E in the treatment of this problem were so successful that many researchers stopped using a "control" group in their studies and simply treated all premature infants with vitamin E, which seems to offer complete protection. The vitamin also shortens the time necessary for the treatment.

Not only can the hyaline membrane of the lung be oxidized during oxygen therapy, but the delicate tissue behind the lens of the eye is also vulnerable. When this tissue oxidizes, it becomes opaque, leads to detachment from the retina, and halts the growth of the eyes. Some of the same doctors who found vitamin E's benefit in BPD have also reported that the vitamin also protects infants from RLF. One even remarked that vitamin E therapy should be routine even for premature infants not given oxygen, since room air itself has oxygen concentrations *twice* that of the uterus.[46]

Although most of the researchers appeared to use injections of vitamin E in their treatment of newborns, Canadian doctors have found that premature infants can absorb vitamin E given orally. Other researchers, however, *have* found impaired absorption of the vitamin in premature infants.[47]

Low vitamin E levels have been found to be a factor in the development of neonatal jaundice, or bilirubinemia, which results from the destruction of too many red blood cells. Injections of the vitamin can help correct this problem.[48] Children with malabsorption of dietary fats have also been found to benefit from vitamin E therapy.[49]

Vitamin E and Breast Cysts

A Baltimore doctor has found that vitamin E supplements (600 IU per day) can produce a "good clinical response" in women with fibrocystic breast disease. When the women were taken off supplementary vitamin E, their cysts returned. Although these cysts are noncancerous, there is a much higher incidence of breast cancer in women who have cysts. Vitamin

E is thought to affect the cysts by increasing adrenal hormone production. It is this corrected hormone balance that doctors feel may help prevent breast cancer, too.[50]

Vitamin E and the Pill

Oral contraceptives are known to lower blood concentrations of vitamin E. One of the side effects of the Pill is thrombosis (blood clots), and there may be a connection between the vitamin E deficiency and this increased tendency for the blood to clot. When doctors have given vitamin E supplements (1200 IU) to women on the Pill, their platelet count has fallen, indicating that the vitamin *is* diminishing the tendency of their blood to clot.[51]

Vitamin E and Osteoarthritis

An Israeli study found that vitamin E may help relieve pain in osteoarthritis. Thirty-two patients were given either vitamin E (600 IU a day) or a placebo for ten days, and then switched. More than half (fifty-two percent) of the people experienced marked relief of pain when taking the supplements of vitamin E, yet only one person did so when taking the placebo. The doctors believe vitamin E's anti-inflammatory effect is due to its stabilizing effect on the membranes of the cells.[52]

Vitamin E and Autoimmune Diseases

Autoimmune diseases are disorders of the body's immune system. Instead of attacking only infectious organisms and foreign substances, the immune system attacks normal tissue which it believes to be foreign. There is some evidence that these autoinflammations are caused by peroxidation of the cell membranes, which releases enzymes which denature normal tissue proteins and converts them into foreign tissues (as far as the immune system is concerned). Antibodies are produced, which attack the tissue.

Two California doctors have been successfully treating several autoimmune diseases with high doses of vitamin E. These include *porphyria cutanea tarda* (1200 to 1600 IU daily), *discoid lupus erythematosus* (900 to 1600 IU daily), *scleroderma* (800 to 1200 IU daily), *morphea* (800 to 1200 IU daily), *Raynaud's Phenomenon* (800 to 1200 IU daily), *vasculitis* (800 to 1600 IU daily), and *polymyositis* (1600 IU daily).

Vitamin E and Muscular Dystrophy

Vitamin E supplementation has been shown to promote significant repair of muscles damaged by nutritional muscular dystrophy in animals. Vitamin E reversed the dystrophic process and stimulated the removal of dead fibers and the return of normal muscle tissue structure.[54] No reports of the use of vitamin E in human muscular dystrophy are evident, however.

Vitamin E and Cystic Fibrosis

Studies have shown that many, if not all, people with cystic fibrosis of the pancreas have deficient blood levels of vitamin E. This disease causes malabsorption of dietary fats. Since vitamin E is a fat-soluble vitamin, a deficiency might almost be expected. Supplementation of CF patients with water-miscible vitamin E (400 IU daily) resulted in normal blood levels of the vitamin. Before supplementation, all the CF patients had subclinical evidence of shortened lifespan of their red blood cells. The vitamin supplementation corrected this. The doctors who conducted the study recommended vitamin E supplements for all people with CF and other malabsorption syndromes.[55]

Vitamin E and Sickle Cell Anemia

Vitamin E has been found to be low in people with sickle cell anemia. Sickled red blood cells have also been found to be especially susceptible to oxidation. In one study, vitamin E (450 IU a day) was given to people with sickle cell anemia. Their red blood cells were then examined. Not only did the supplementation raise their vitamin E concentrations to normal or above normal, but it also cut to less than half the number of irreversibly sickled cells in their blood. The researchers did not test whether or not vitamin E supplements would have any effects on the clinical symptoms of sickle cell anemia.[56]

Vitamin E and Periodontal Health

Vitamin E has shown effectiveness in reducing tartar on the teeth and inflammation of the gums. A British dentist found that eighty percent of his patients with a tartar problem who took supplemental doses of vitamin E returned after six months with markedly less tartar.[57] Daily supplements of 800 IU of vitamin E have been shown to reduce inflammation of the gums, as measured by gingival exudate. Researchers believe that vitamin E reduces the hormone-induced (prostaglandin) inflammatory response.[58]

Vitamin E and Genetic Defects

Vitamin E may prove to be a successful treatment for one of the commonest genetic defects, the G6PD deficiency, which afflicts about ten percent of black males and between three and eight percent of males of Mediterranean origins—all told, about 100 million people across the world. G6PD deficiency causes a serious, sometimes fatal, reaction to chemicals in aspirin, sulfa drugs, chloramphenicol, chloroquine, and fava beans. The chemical causes increased oxidation of the cell membranes of the red blood cells. Doctors in the United States have tried high doses of vitamin E (800 IU) on a child with the disease, and the anemia caused by the defect was significantly reduced.[59]

Another defect in the maintenance of the red blood cells is

thalassemia. Mediterranean people are also more susceptible to this inherited defect, in which the red blood cells become too brittle to survive. Vitamin E has been shown to restore near-normal resilience to weakened red blood cells in this disease.[60]

HOW MUCH VITAMIN E DO WE NEED?

In 1974 the RDA for vitamin E was *lowered* from a maximum of 30 IU to 15 IU. It *now* stands at 10 IU for men and 8 IU for women. The primary reason for the drop seems to be that dieticians were complaining that it was difficult, if not impossible, to compose diets which supplied 30 IU of vitamin E. That's not surprising when you understand that refining of flour removes just about *all* of the vitamin E. White flour products devoid of vitamin E (since the vitamin is not replaced by fortification) make up a sizeable portion of the calories in the average diet. Several authorities on vitamin E, including the researcher who performed the only human deficiency study, have stated that the new RDA is too low to maintain adequate vitamin E status.[61]

Many surveys indicate that large numbers of people are not receiving adequate vitamin E in their diets. The blood concentration necessary to prevent excess oxidative damage to the red blood cells is about 1 mg. per 100 ml. of blood. Yet concentrations of less than half this amount have been found in approximately one percent of the Canadian population and in six percent of Canadian university students. Surveys of American diets reveal that the average vitamin E consumption is about 11 to 13 IU, with many daily intakes below 3 IU.[62]

Many factors can contribute to a vitamin E deficiency. Polyunsaturated fatty acids in the diet can raise requirements for the vitamin in two ways. First of all, vitamin E is required to protect the unsaturated fatty acids in the cells and membranes. The higher the concentrations of these substances in the diet, the higher will be their concentrations in the tissues. Therefore, that much more vitamin E will be needed to prevent oxidation. Polyunsaturated fatty acids also appear to interfere with vitamin E in the intestine, whether by competing for absorption or through some other mechanism. Doctors have calculated that for every gram of polyunsaturated fatty acids in the diet, an additional 1 IU of vitamin E is required to prevent a subclinical deficiency.[63] Since a great many people are using more and more polyunsaturated oils in their diets, the potential number of subclinical vitamin E deficiencies is tremendous.

Other factors can interfere with the metabolism of vitamin E and raise requirements. One of these, apparently, is supplemental *iron*. It was once thought that iron and vitamin E blocked the absorption of each other in the intestines, but it is now thought that their reaction is at the cellular level. Animals and humans deficient in vitamin E are more vulnerable to iron toxicity than when vitamin E is adequate or supplemental. In trials with premature infants, it was found that routine iron supplements were toxic because the infants were deficient in vitamin E. Giving them extra vitamin E prevented toxic reactions to iron. This "destruction" of vitamin E by supplemental iron has not been fully explained. It may be that iron encourages the oxidation of the red blood cells unless enough vitamin E is present to prevent it. Supplemental iron does produce excess oxidative destruction of red blood cells when vitamin E levels are low.[64] Since many diets don't provide enough *iron* as well as vitamin E, this should not be taken as a suggestion not to take iron supplements. Many people need iron supplements. This evidence does suggest, however, that people who do take iron supplements should perhaps also take vitamin E.

Since vitamin E is a fat-soluble vitamin, ingestion of mineral oil or laxatives can also interfere with its absorption. Smoking has also been shown to increase oxidative stress on body tissues, thus raising vitamin E requirements. Estrogens in oral contraceptives and menopausal drugs also cause a vitamin E deficiency. Studies have found that women on the

Pill have only forty to fifty-six percent as much vitamin E in their blood as women not taking oral contraceptives.[65] Hyperthyroidism has also been shown to increase vitamin E needs.[66]

TOXICITY OF VITAMIN E

Although it is a fat-soluble vitamin and stored in the body, vitamin E does not appear to be toxic. As for side effects, there was a report of muscular weakness in one person taking vitamin E supplements, but no other researcher or doctor has reported a similar effect, including those who have looked for it in their patients taking supplements.[67] A study of vitamin E supplementation in 202 healthy college students found that 600 IU of vitamin E daily caused no muscular weakness or gastrointestinal upset, but that there was a reduction in thyroid hormone levels and, in women, an increase in blood levels of triglycerides. No symptoms resulted from these biochemical changes.[68] Other studies have found that high doses of vitamin E can also lower the basal metabolism rate and slightly increase blood fats. Some studies have found, however, that vitamin E can lower cholesterol, too.

Most studies, including those finding some biochemical changes with vitamin E supplementation, find no significant adverse or harmful effects from vitamin E.[69] Doses up to 1600 IU have been used for prolonged periods of time without harm. Of course, people with bleeding disorders should use vitamin E cautiously and only under a doctor's supervision, since vitamin E "thins" the blood. People already taking anticoagulant drugs should also be aware that they might thin their blood too much.[70] Doctors also caution against the use of high doses of vitamin E in cases of high blood pressure, congestive heart failure, badly damaged heart, and insulin-dependent diabetes. In these cases, they recommend starting out with low doses (100 IU) when supplementation is required.[71] People with underactive thyroid taking thyroid hormone may find that vitamin E reduces the effectiveness of the drug.[72]

SOURCES OF VITAMIN E

The richest natural sources of vitamin E are the oils in the seeds of cereal grains. Wheat germ oil is foremost among these, followed by soybean oil, cottonseed oil, sunflower seed oil, and corn oil. Nuts, eggs, fish, and organ meats contribute considerably smaller quantities. Because fruits and vegetables are not consumed in the quantities necessary to provide enough vitamin E, they are not considered significant sources.

There is more than one form of vitamin E, or tocopherol. Actually, there are at least *four* tocopherols which have been isolated, the *alpha*, *beta*, *gamma*, and *delta* tocopherols. Of the four, the alpha fraction is the most active, and in vitamin E supplements the level of vitamin E activity (international units, IU) is measured according to how much *alpha tocopherol* is present. Synthetic vitamin E is synthetic alpha tocopherol. In vitamin supplements, the natural form of vitamin E will be labeled d-alpha tocopherol, and the synthetic dl-alpha tocopherol. The natural form of vitamin E is more potent; however, this difference in potency is accounted for in calculating vitamin E "activity" in IU. So a supplement of 100 IU of d-alpha will be as potent as 100 IU of dl-alpha tocopherol. One researcher did find that the natural form and the water-soluble form of vitamin E were more effective in raising blood levels than the synthetic form. But this was measured in persons with lupus erythematosus. No such comparison is available for healthy persons.[73] For most of the studies and therapeutic uses described, the standard form of vitamin E is the synthetic form.

Cooking does not normally destroy significant amounts of vitamin E. Frying, however, especially in deep fat, can cause most of the vitamin E to be oxidized. Storage for long periods can destroy vitamin E, too.

Vitamin E supplements are available in doses ranging from a few IU to over 1000 IU.

16

Vitamin K

Vitamin K gets its name from the Scandinavian word *koagulation*, which means the same as its English counterpart, coagulation. In this case, the name is an indication of the function. Vitamin K is essential to the formation of precursors of thrombin, which is the active agent in the clotting of blood. Thrombin acts upon fibrinogen to form the fibrin blood clot. Vitamin K does not actually become part of the clot or the precursors of thrombin, though it is required for their synthesis in the liver.

A deficiency of vitamin K results in lowered levels of prothrombin and other precursors of thrombin, and, therefore, reduced coagulability of the blood and increased bleeding tendency. Recent research suggests that vitamin K is also necessary for other biochemical functions besides coagulation. Animal studies have shown it is required for proper bone mineralization.[1]

Vitamin K deficiency is relatively rare because the vitamin is

184

synthesized by intestinal bacteria. However, in newborns vitamin K deficiency is fairly common, if not the rule, since newborns have no intestinal bacteria. If the deficiency is severe enough, bleeding from the gastrointestinal tract, bloody stools, or bloody vomiting occur within the first week or so of life. Internal bleeding or bleeding from the umbilicus can follow. In adults, vitamin K deficiency can result in excess bleeding from wounds and blood in the urine and stools.

There is no RDA for vitamin K, since authorities feel a deficiency of the vitamin is not possible under normal conditions.

Nevertheless, deficiencies do exist. Many common factors can cause a vitamin K deficiency. Antibiotic therapy is the most common cause of a deficiency. The vitamin-producing bacteria in the gut are destroyed by antibiotics, thus removing the primary source of this vitamin. Diet can also be a factor. In a study of thirteen hospital patients with vitamin K-deficiency bleeding disorders, all thirteen were nutritionally deficient while ten of the thirteen were receiving antibiotics. These researchers reported vitamin K deficiency in at least .05 percent (one in 2000) of *all* patients admitted to their hospitals over a two-year period. However, among the patients referred for bleeding disorders, 2.3 percent had vitamin K deficiencies.[2]

Another doctor found twenty-two vitamin K deficiencies among surgical patients, then decided to measure vitamin K status in all patients in the hospital surgical and medical wards. He found twenty-seven more vitamin K-deficient people. Twenty-two of them were receiving antibiotics, while nineteen were receiving no food through the mouth. The rest had poor diets, too. This doctor estimated the number of gastrointestinal surgery patients developing vitamin K deficiency in the hospital was .4 percent (four in every 1000) and .08 percent (four in 5000) among hospital patients in general. He also stated that he felt his estimates were probably low.[3]

Besides antibiotics, sulfa drugs can lead to a vitamin K deficiency. Anticoagulant drugs often work by interfering with vitamin K. And vitamin K deficiency hemorrhaging can occur in newborns born to epileptic mothers taking barbiturates or phenytoin.[4] Since vitamin K is a fat-soluble vitamin, any drug or disorder which interferes with absorption of fat will impair vitamin K absorption. Some of these conditions are pancreatic dysfunction, sprue, celiac disease, steatorrhea, and ingestion of mineral oil.

SOURCES OF VITAMIN K

The richest natural sources of vitamin K are the green leafy vegetables, such as cabbage, cauliflower, and spinach. Liver and soybeans are also good sources. Of course, the primary source is synthesis by bacteria in the intestine.

Vitamin K is not destroyed by heat, but it is vulnerable to oxidation, acids, alkali, and light.

Although there is no reported toxicity for natural vitamin K in adults, the vitamin is available in supplemental form only through a doctor's prescription.

section 2
MINERALS

17

Calcium

Imagine you've just moved into the dream house you designed yourself. You've built lots of exposed beams, real hardwood floors, walnut paneling, pine cabinets, cedar closets, oak countertops in the kitchen and bar, a cedar shake roof, and a woodstove for heat.

What would happen if vandals dumped a bucket of hungry termites in your cellar? If you found out about it soon enough, you'd call the exterminator, who would come out right away and try to eliminate the problem.

But what if you didn't go down into your cellar all that often and it was a month or two before you discovered the infestation? Not only would the exterminator's visit cost quite a bit more, but your chances of completely eliminating the termites would be severely diminished.

What if you hardly ever went into your cellar? What if the infestation went completely undiscovered for month after month after month? Then, to celebrate your first year in your dream house you threw a great party, invited all your friends, really tried to stretch the rafters.

You and your guests might be in for a surprise. Those floor beams and rafters and panels and walls and countertops and doors and stairs that have been eaten away by termites for a year might hold up fine when there's only you to stress them. But when you and your party start to boogie, your whole house may collapse like so many balsa wood sticks!

This is exactly what can happen to your body if you allow your calcium supply to fall behind the demand. Every day your body doesn't get enough calcium is like a bucket of termites going unnoticed in your skeletal "basement." And just like a frame house that's been infested with termites, your bones will be weakened by holes and pits where calcium should be.

You might not notice the "infestation" until it's too late— until your skeletal structure collapses under the excess stress of a "party." Something as simple as a missed step on the way downstairs could land you in the hospital for a season. Or a slip on the ski slope could wrap up your winter career for some time to come. Or your dentist could one day break the bad news that you're losing some teeth because your jaw has been losing calcium for a decade or two. And you haven't had the slightest indication of what's been happening.

WHAT CALCIUM DOES

Calcium is the main structural mineral in the body. About ninety-nine percent of the body's three pounds of calcium is in the skeleton and teeth and is responsible for their hardness and strength. Calcium in the bones and teeth is not *permanently* stationed there, because the bones and teeth also serve as a *reservoir* for calcium. There is an almost constant exchange of calcium between the bones and the body fluids and soft tissues, where the rest of the calcium is located. Because the body's homeostatic mechanism maintains relatively constant blood levels of calcium, if dietary intake does not make up for what is lost through excretion, what is taken from the bones will not be replaced.

That one percent of the body's calcium outside the skeleton is also very important. It is essential for the strength of the intracellular membranes and for many important enzyme reactions involved in the clotting of blood and other processes; it regulates the excitability of peripheral nerves and muscles so that irritability is increased when calcium is low. Normal muscular contraction and relaxation, including the rhythm of the heart, depend on calcium.

Naturally, calcium is vitally important for growth and development. During the last trimester of pregnancy, between 200 and 300 mg. of calcium is deposited every day in the skeleton of the fetus. Breast milk contains from 250 to 500 mg. of calcium each day. If a pregnant or lactating mother isn't supplying this calcium in her diet, most of it is going to come out of her bones, and the bone health of both mother and child will suffer.

Since the body maintains fairly constant blood levels of calcium, low levels occur only in very severe deficiencies. When a deficiency is that bad, muscle spasms and convulsions usually occur. Researchers use what is called calcium "balance" to measure a person's calcium status. The total intake of calcium is measured and compared to the total amount excreted through the urine, feces, and sweat. When the amount excreted is about the same as that ingested, calcium balance is zero, or even. When more calcium is excreted than ingested, calcium balance is negative. And when more calcium is ingested than is excreted, balance is positive.

The balance method is far from perfect, expecially since many factors can affect calcium retention and excretion. But when researchers are careful to eliminate or account for as many of these factors as possible, and when the tests are done over a fairly long period, calcium balance can be a good indicator of whether a person is getting enough calcium in the diet.

Another method is to actually measure and compare the

density of the bones over various lengths of time. This method, of course, is the best way to find out if enough calcium is being supplied in the diet, because if the diet is deficient, the bones lose calcium and become less dense.

Insufficient dietary calcium can be a factor in rickets, osteomalacia, and osteoporosis. (See Vitamin D chapter for discussion of rickets and osteomalacia.)

Besides its effects on bone mineralization and nerve and muscle irritability, calcium deficiency can also affect blood and tissue levels of two poisonous metals, lead and cadmium. When dietary calcium is low, the body retains more lead. This has been demonstrated in several experiments with both humans and animals: low dietary calcium causes high blood and tissue levels of lead.[1]

Low dietary calcium actually causes animals to *eat more* lead. Calcium deficient rats and monkeys voluntarily consume up to *forty-four times* the amount of lead via lead-containing water than they will under normal circumstances, even when pure water is available. Injecting the animals with toxic levels of lead still does not erase or diminish their preference for lead.[2] Since human studies have demonstrated that children deficient in calcium also have higher blood levels of lead, there appears to be a connection between lead poisoning and calcium deficiency. The real villain in lead poisoning may not be lead in paint, but inadequate diet.

Cadmium, another toxic pollutant, is also retained by the body in higher concentrations when calcium is low.[3]

Calcium and Osteoporosis

Osteoporosis can be caused by a diet deficient in calcium and vitamin D, and the gradual loss of bone minerals which occurs in osteoporosis can be inhibited, halted, or *reversed* by adequate calcium and vitamin D supplementation.

Osteoporosis is an insidious disease; the symptoms are usually not apparent until the disease is in the advanced stages. In many cases, the progressive weakening of the bones, as porous gaps develop where minerals are removed, first shows up when bones of the hip, spine, or limbs simply *break spontaneously, with no stress but normal weight-bearing*. In some people, especially postmenopausal women, low back pain is the first symptom. Loss of bone mass in the spine eventually results in shortening of height and the "dowager's hump."

Current estimates are that more than 14,000,000 women are visibly affected by osteoporosis in the United States.[4] This is not to say that men and other women are not affected in some way. *We all lose minerals from our bones.* The difference is that men can start losing bone density between the ages of forty-five and fifty-five, while in women the process starts about ten years *earlier*.[5] In the United States, more than one-third of the over a million fractures which occur in women over forty-five every year are associated with osteoporosis.[6] Other studies have found a similar close correlation between bone density and hip, vertebral, and long-limb fractures in women. Osteoporosis severe enough to cause fractures is estimated to occur in at least ten percent of men and women over fifty.[7]

The first bone where demineralization usually occurs is the jaw bone.[8] When tooth-bearing bone is lost, the result is periodontal disease. Like osteoporosis, periodontal disease is insidious. It begins at a relatively early age and progresses many years before teeth are loosened and finally lost. Almost eighty percent of the people in the United States have some degree of periodontal disease, and fully half have lost teeth to the disease by the age of sixty. Periodontal disease, of course, involves many symptoms besides loss of minerals from the jaw bone. Nevertheless, progressive loss of alveolar (jaw) bone and detachment of teeth have been associated with calcium deficiency or imbalance and osteoporosis in other areas of the body.[9]

The question is whether correcting the calcium deficiency can inhibit or possibly *reverse* the loss of bone density. Several studies have answered this question in the affirmative. Doctors and dentists from Cornell Medical College and the University of Gothenburg, Sweden, gave 500 mg. supplements of calcium (in the form of calcium gluconolactate and calcium carbonate) twice a day to ten people with periodontal disease. The daily diet was found to contain only 200 to 350 mg. of calcium in nine of the ten people (one person had a daily intake of 850 mg.). After six months of supplementation, symptoms such as bleeding gums, gingivitis, and loose teeth either disappeared or were remarkably reduced. Bone loss was stopped, and in seven out of ten people, was *reversed:* bone density *increased* in the tooth-bearing bone.[10]

Another group of researchers confirmed that low dietary calcium levels lead to resorption of alveolar bone, and went on to test the effects of daily supplements of 750 mg. of calcium (calcium carbonate) plus vitamin D (375 units) on people who had already lost teeth because of bone demineralization. Bone density was not increased in this trial, but loss of density was *reduced* by thirty-four to thirty-nine percent.[11]

Can calcium supplementation do the same for bones in other parts of the body? Apparently. Dr. Anthony Albanese and his colleagues at the Burke Rehabilitation Center in White Plains, New York, have performed many trials with calcium supplements in osteoporosis. In one study, twelve elderly women between the ages of seventy-nine and eighty-nine were given supplements of 750 mg. of calcium plus 375 units of vitamin D. After three years of supplementation, the average bone density of the group *increased* by six percent. In a matched group of women who were not supplemented, bone density decreased by seven percent.

Dr. Albanese then tried calcium supplements on a group of younger women (ages thirty-six to sixty-two). No changes in bone density were measured during the first six to nine months. After that, however, changes started to occur, dramatically in some women, slowly and steadily in others. After three years of supplementation, bone density in six (out of fourteen) women rose to the level found in men of similar ages. One of the women stopped taking supplements, and within a year her bone density fell from well above the normal level for her age to *below* normal.

Many doctors maintain that the reason women start to lose bone density is the reduction in hormone levels that begins around the menopause. This is a controversial point, because women are known to lose bone density even *before* estrogen levels start to drop. Nevertheless, the standard treatment for menopausal osteoporosis in many doctor's offices is still estrogen supplements.

Dr. Albanese and his colleagues conducted a study in which the effects of calcium supplements were compared to the effect of estrogen supplements. One group of women received calcium alone; one received calcium plus estrogen; one received estrogen alone; and one received placebo pills. The women who received calcium alone or calcium with estrogen did experience increased bone density. But the women who received a placebo or estrogen alone continued to lose bone. Dr. Albanese went on to study bone density and fracture risk in women who were taking estrogen supplements, and found that calcium intake, more than estrogen, was the predicting factor in bone density and fracture risk.[12]

Studies by other researchers have confirmed Dr. Albanese's success in halting or reversing loss of bone density because of inadequate calcium in the diet.[13]

One other factor seems to be involved in osteoporosis, one which no amount of supplementation can take the place of, and that is *exercise*. Bone loss occurs in both men and women whenever exercise or physical activity is severely reduced. Even the *astronauts* were found to lose bone density during space flights when exercise programs were insufficient. It doesn't require extended periods of inactivity to cause bone loss, because the astronauts started losing significant amounts of calcium after only three days.[14] One study demonstrated that as little as one hour of exercise three times a week resulted in an *increase* in bone density in eighteen postmenopausal women.[15]

A study of the biochemical effects of exercise helped explain this phenomenon by showing that exercise increased blood levels of calcium and affected certain hormone levels in such a way as to favor maintenance of bone density.[16] Other studies have shown that skeletal mass is usually higher in runners.[17] And finally, one study revealed that even among men and women of college student age (twenty to twenty-five), variations in bone density were associated with levels of physical activity *and* amount of calcium in the diet.

So it appears that even young adults can reduce their chances of developing osteoporosis later in life, and that men and women of all ages should make sure they have enough calcium in their diets *and* enough physical activity in their lives.[18]

Calcium and Heart Disease

Several studies have uncovered evidence that calcium may play a role in heart disease prevention and treatment. One of Dr. Albanese's trials with calcium supplements (750 mg. per day) found that not only was bone density maintained or increased by supplements, but blood levels of *cholesterol* were also reduced. Dr. Albanese also cited other studies in which calcium supplements were found to lower blood concentrations of both cholesterol and triglycerides by as much as twenty-five percent. Another study found that calcium specifically lowered the LDL cholesterol (the cholesterol which is on its way *into* the tissues).[19]

Calcium also plays an important role in platelet function; however, no research has as yet shown that calcium deficiency will adversely affect blood clotting in such a way as to cause a thrombus or embolism. But in animal studies, calcium apparently lessened many of the damaging effects of oxygen deprivation on the heart muscle.

Some studies have even shown that in communities with hard water (which will be higher in calcium), the death rate from cardiovascular disease is lower than in communities with soft water. In a British study, towns which had switched from hard water to soft water experienced a rise in cardiovascular disease over a thirty-year period, whereas towns which had switched to hard water from soft experienced a decrease in the disease.[20] Such information, however, should not be interpreted on too simple a level. There are many different factors in the differences between hard water and soft water that may have an effect on cardiovascular disease. Hard water is richer in many minerals besides calcium, whereas soft water often contains some potentially toxic metals in greater quantity than hard water. If anything, this information suggests that we shouldn't be too hasty in equipping our water supplies with softeners, since softening the water may eventually harden the arteries.

REQUIREMENTS FOR CALCIUM

The RDA for calcium ranges from a low of 360 mg. for infants to a high of 1200 mg. for pregnant and lactating women. The RDA for adults, both men and women, is 800 mg. Of all the RDAs, this is perhaps the most controversial. Earlier publications by the National Research Council even contained arguments as to why the requirement should be raised or lowered. Finally, so much pressure was put on the committee that set the RDA that the arguments were *dropped* from future publications. Some members wanted to lower the RDA to as low as 600 mg. The significance of the removal of the pro and con arguments is that the controversy was effectively denied.[21]

The controversy did not go away, however. Nature does not obey the committee and change biochemical reality to suit the RDA. Many of the researchers whose studies have been cited have found not only that *the RDA of 800 mg. is not enough to maintain positive calcium balance, but also that few women (or men) are even getting the RDA.* The doctors from Cornell who found that calcium supplements reversed alveolar bone loss stated that the average loss of calcium through excretion totals 380 mg. per day. To maintain positive calcium balance, at least that much must be resupplied through the diet. However, all the calcium that is eaten is not absorbed. The average amount, they say, is thirty-five percent. So in order to replace the average daily losses, almost 1100 mg. of calcium would have to be supplied every day. Of course, the amount of calcium absorbed is not always thirty-five percent; it can range from two percent to forty percent. So even 1100 mg. might not be enough for many people.[22]

Another group of doctors tested calcium balance in 130 healthy women aged thirty-five to fifty. They found that women with the higher calcium intakes also had higher calcium balances. On the average, however, the women were not receiving the RDA of calcium in their diets, and their calcium balances were negative. *But even the women with calcium intake above the RDA had negative calcium balances.*

On the basis of these figures, the doctors concluded that it would take a daily calcium intake of at least fifty percent greater than the RDA to maintain a zero balance, and that this amount (1241 mg.) *could* be too low for *at least half the women.* Obviously, the current RDA is not adequate for very much of the population.[23]

An orthopedic researcher from the Mayo Clinic has reported that calcium absorption begins to diminish at age *twenty* and that bone loss begins at age *twenty-five*, and that supplementation should probably begin at that age to avoid osteoporosis.[24]

The USDA found that consumption of calcium is generally thirty percent below the RDA in women over thirty-five. In women over forty-five, the average amount consumed was only 450 mg.—*almost fifty percent less than the RDA.* Dr. Albanese and other researchers have clearly established that this amount is not sufficient to prevent loss of bone density.[25] Since calcium absorption becomes less efficient the older we get, it's no wonder osteoporosis is considered by many to be "normal" with advancing age.

Many other factors can contribute to a calcium deficiency. A high-protein diet, for example, causes more calcium to be excreted, thus raising the amount needed to maintain a positive calcium balance. High-fiber foods have been found to reduce calcium absorption. A small amount of fat in the intestine seems to improve calcium absorption; however, an excess of fat may form insoluble calcium soaps and sharply reduce absorption. Recent studies have also shown that refined sugar (white sugar) causes a sharp increase in calcium excretion.[26]

Several common drugs and over-the-counter medications inhibit calcium absorption or utilization. These include antacids, tetracycline antibiotics, laxatives, diuretics, heparin, and anticonvulsant drugs.[27]

The most common factor in calcium absorption and utilization is the ratio of calcium to phosphorus in the diet. There is a consensus among most researchers that too much phosphorus in the diet can adversely affect calcium balance. They recommend a calcium-to-phosphorus ratio in the diet of 1:1 for adults (equal calcium and phosphorus) and *greater* than 1:1 for children, pregnant women, and nursing mothers. They cite evidence that a ratio less than one (more phosphorus than calcium) will cause increased excretion of calcium.[28]

Unfortunately, the average ratio in the American diet is more like 1:2.8. The average American is eating almost *three times* more phosphorus than calcium.[29] And our intake of phosphorus seems to be increasing while our intake of calcium decreases. Many of the most popular foods in the supermarket contain many times more phosphorus than calcium. Most meat, for example, has a calcium-to-phosphorus ratio of 1:20. In case you've ever wondered why they call soda and pop "soft drinks," it's because of their potential for *softening the bones and teeth.* These beverages contain massive amounts of phosphorus. Other processed foods have extra phosphorus added to them in the form of preservatives, dyes, and other cosmetic agents. Processed meats, cheeses, dressings, refrigerated bakery products, and breads are among the foods with added phosphorus.[30]

Furthermore, studies have shown that both the average

college dining hall meal and the average fast-food restaurant meal are deficient in calcium, and that their calcium-phosphorus ratio is much too low.[31]

TOXICITY

None of the studies described in this chapter, or any others encountered while researching this chapter, reported any adverse effects from the levels of supplementation used (750 to 1500 mg.).

SOURCES OF CALCIUM

For a newborn baby, the best source of calcium is mother's milk, which has a calcium-phosphorus ratio of 2.4:1. Cow's milk, with a ratio of 1.2:1, is a good source for everyone else, but is not the only good natural source of calcium. Egg yolk, fish (eaten with the *bones*), soybeans, green leafy vegetables such as turnip greens, mustard greens, broccoli, and kale; roots, tubers, and seeds; and stews and soups made with bones can provide considerable calcium.[32] Lactose (the sugar found in milk and milk products) has a positive effect on calcium absorption.

Supplements of calcium are available in many forms (calcium carbonate, calcium gluconate, calcium lactate, etc.). There is no general agreement over which form is the best. It is probably wise to use more than one form in a supplement program. (Don't forget that vitamin D also is necessary for calcium absorption and utilization.) Calcium supplements are available in a wide range of dose levels, from less than 100 mg. to several hundred milligrams.

18

Chromium

If the shiny chrome bumpers fall off your car, the car will still function as well as it did before. Chromium is not very important to an automobile's performance. In fact, the car may perform *better* without lugging around the many pounds of chrome as dead weight.

In the body's "engine," it's a different story: a few hundred *micrograms* of chromium can make *all* the difference in how efficiently the body burns its fuel. And that can make a big difference in how close to optimum health you are, since every life function, from walking and talking to thinking and sleeping, depends on that part of the metabolism which renders fuel sugar from carbohydrates and makes it available to the cells for burning.

WHAT CHROMIUM DOES

Insulin, of course, is the hormone which regulates the

body's burning of sugar. Insulin doesn't do the job alone, however. Chromium helps. Without chromium, insulin can't do the job at all. In addition to its role as cofactor for insulin, chromium also plays a role in the metabolism of fats, proteins, and nucleic acids (DNA, RNA).

The first hints that chromium was essential to the body's metabolism of sugar came in 1955, when researchers found that rats maintained on a diet of torula yeast (*not* brewer's yeast) had impaired glucose tolerance: their bodies could not handle very large doses of sugar. No other nutrients could overcome this deficit, so the researchers concluded that something was *missing* from the torula yeast. They named this mystery substance Glucose Tolerance Factor, or GTF. Subsequently, GTF was found to exist in brewer's yeast, and the active principal was identified as trivalent chromium (other forms of chromium are toxic). Further experiments with chromium revealed that a severe deficiency caused impaired glucose tolerance as serious as mild diabetes, and corneal opacities.

Chromium deficiency has also been found to raise blood levels of cholesterol and produce a high incidence of plaques on the aorta (main artery from the heart). Chromium may also be a cofactor for certain parts of the protein transport process. And high concentrations of chromium are found in nucleic acids, leading investigators to speculate that chromium is important in their synthesis, too. In animals, low-chromium diets result in depression of growth rate, shortened life span, and reduced ability to withstand stress. Adding *extra* chromium to animals' drinking water, however, resulted in higher growth rates and sharply reduced death rates. In fact, the chromium-supplemented mice and rats set *records for longevity* by living an average of ninety-nine days longer than the animals not receiving chromium supplements. Furthermore, the supplemented rats and mice were free of aortic plaques, while twenty percent of the unsupplemented rats had such lesions, though they were supposed to be receiving "adequate" chromium.[1]

Chromium and Glucose Intolerance

In *1853*, a British physician reported using brewer's yeast to successfully treat a case of diabetes. After a little more than six weeks on brewer's yeast (one tablespoon, two to three times a day, in milk), the patient stopped urinating sugar and regained his original weight. A modern doctor examining this case concluded that the patient's diabetes was caused by a chromium deficiency, which the brewer's yeast corrected.[2]

Several recent studies have revealed that chromium, or GTF, may indeed help many people with glucose intolerance. Many of the symptoms of chromium deficiency are identical to diabetes. Tests have shown that people with impaired glucose tolerance have an increased need for chromium.[3] Protein-calorie malnutrition is often accompanied by impaired glucose tolerance (inability to remove sugar from the blood and utilize it) and fasting hypoglycemia (a state of chronic low blood levels of sugar). Studies with children in Jordan, Nigeria, Turkey, and Egypt have shown that chromium supplements can bring about "spectacular" improvements in glucose tolerance. Researchers feel that a protein deficiency worsens the effects of a chromium deficiency.

Tests of adults with glucose intolerance have also shown that chromium deficiency is often a factor. In one study, three out of six people with mild diabetes improved their glucose tolerance by taking chromium supplements (180 to 1000 micrograms) for seven to thirteen weeks. In another study, four out of ten people with diabetic glucose tolerance were restored to *normal* glucose tolerance with supplements of 150 micrograms of chromium daily. The people who responded tended to have milder impairments of glucose tolerance. Fifty percent of a group of middle-aged people with impaired glucose tolerance responded to chromium supplementation (150 micrograms) with improved tolerance. One thousand micrograms daily brought improvement to four out of twelve diabetics, while 150 micrograms failed to have any effect in sixteen others, in another study.[4] And doctors report that diabetics have been able to reduce their insulin requirements by including brewer's yeast in their daily diets.[5]

CAN EXTRA CHROMIUM DO ANY GOOD?

Some researchers have interpreted such responses to chromium by stating that chromium potentiates or "spares" insulin, meaning it makes insulin metabolism more efficient. Although it's generally accepted that a chromium deficiency will impair glucose tolerance and that correcting the deficiency will improve or restore it, it is still a matter of controversy whether or not *extra* chromium will result in better-than-normal glucose tolerance and carbohydrate metabolism. Some of the animal experiments already described seem to suggest that extra chromium *does* have a boosting effect on certain factors. And a recent study of people with normal and impaired glucose tolerance found that chromium supplements seemed to have an insulin-sparing effect on normal people, too.[6]

Of course, this doesn't necessarily mean that taking chromium supplements will change your life in any way, unless you have glucose intolerance. It may only suggest that most people are not getting *enough* chromium, but that the effects on glucose tolerance are not always apparent or even measurable except by very precise biochemical tests.

Chromium and Heart Disease

It is really impossible to separate a discussion of chromium and diabetes from chromium and heart disease, especially since the leading cause of death among diabetics is cardiovascular disease. The link between impaired glucose tolerance and cardiovascular disease has been well established. And many of the studies which demonstrate chromium's role in cardiovascular disease are also relevant to impaired glucose tolerance. In animals, of course, the link is pretty clear:

chromium-deficient animals have impaired glucose tolerance *and* atherosclerotic plaques in their aortas.

In humans, the links are there too. Dr. Henry Schroeder, one of the leading trace mineral researchers, has found that not only do diabetics suffer the lesions of atherosclerosis, but that people with atherosclerosis also have impaired glucose tolerance, which chromium supplements can improve. Dr. Schroeder has also used chromium supplements to lower blood levels of cholesterol by as much as twenty-six percent.[7]

Other researchers have confirmed Dr. Schroeder's findings and revealed new connections. A study in which chromium supplements (from yeast) were given to twenty-seven women, aged forty to seventy-five, found that not only did glucose tolerance improve in those who were hyperglycemic (too much sugar in the blood), but that blood levels of cholesterol were lowered substantially and levels of triglycerides were lowered twelve percent.[8]

A further link between low-chromium status and cardiovascular disease has been found by comparing chromium concentrations in blood, tissue, and aortas among people who have the disease and in healthy people. Aorta concentrations of chromium are lower (or *absent*) in people dying from atherosclerotic heart disease than in people dying from accidents. A recent study tested blood levels of chromium in people with heart disease and people without the disease. The people with heart disease had consistently lower chromium status, while *none* of the people with blood chromium concentration above or equal to 5.5 micrograms per liter had the disease. In fact, low chromium levels were found to be *more reliable in predicting atherosclerosis* than high blood levels of cholesterol and triglycerides, and high blood pressure.[9]

Does this mean that chromium deficiency is *the* cause of cardiovascular disease? No more than the evidence in previous chapters means that vitamin C or pyridoxine deficiencies are the cause. Obviously, *all* of these factors contribute. As attractive as the connection between this single nutrient and the disease may seem to be, there are too many additional, and equally attractive, factors to rely on this one *alone*. Don't expect chromium supplementation to make up for deficiencies in other areas that also may contribute to cardiovascular disease.

REQUIREMENTS FOR CHROMIUM

At this time, there is no RDA for chromium, even though many scientists recognize that it is essential. The National Research Council only "suggests" that an intake of .05 to .2 mg. per day is "adequate" and "safe." The reason for this uncertainty is that there is as yet no definitive measurement of the amount of *active* chromium, or GTF, in most foods. This makes it difficult to determine how much an average diet provides and exactly how much chromium *is* required.

Although we don't know exactly how much we need, we do suspect that quite a few people probably aren't getting enough chromium. Dr. Schroeder and his colleagues found that tissue concentrations of chromium in Americans were substantially lower than those in most foreigners tested. Orientals, for example, on the average had five times as much chromium in their tissues as Americans. And while 98.5 percent of the foreigners over fifty still had chromium in their tissues, from fifteen to twenty-three percent of the Americans did not. Dr. Schroeder has also found that wild animals have ten times the chromium concentrations the average American does.[10]

The fact that Americans start out with high levels of chromium which decline rather sharply after age ten suggests that our diet is not providing us with enough of the mineral. Of course, it doesn't take complicated blood or tissue tests to figure this out, since food processing and refining removes almost *all* the chromium from foods which are natural sources of the mineral. Nature has a way of providing nutritional "coverage" in many foods. Since carbohydrates require chromium for their proper metabolism, it would seem "right" that high-carbohydrate foods contain high concentrations of chromium. And that's the way it is—until food processing and refining come along. Refining whole wheat into white flour, for example, removes eighty-three percent of the chromium. Natural sugars, of course, are the most concentrated sources of carbohydrates. They would be expected to tax the glucose tolerance system most of all. And in a "protective" natural order of things, they would also be expected to contain high concentrations of chromium. Which they do. Refining cane and beets into white sugar, however, removes *ninety-two percent* of the chromium.[11]

This situation would be bad enough, but the carbohydrates are *still there* to tax the body's metabolism. And they do, resulting in still further depletion of the body's store of chromium.[12] It's not too difficult to see how a diet high in refined carbohydrates can maintain a vicious cycle leading to an ever-worsening chromium deficiency. In how many people does this deficiency become severe enough to contribute to a case of cardiovascular disease?

Other factors may also contribute to chromium deficiency. A low-protein diet aggravates a chromium deficiency. Inorganic chromium salts (as opposed to the chromium-GTF found in yeast and some other foods) are poorly absorbed compared to GTF chromium. Researchers believe the body must convert inorganic chromium to GTF before it can be effective.[13] It is also believed that some people, such as older people and diabetics, lose the ability to convert inorganic chromium to the active form. This may explain why some people with impaired glucose tolerance don't respond to chromium.[14] This also opens up the possibility for wide variation in human requirements.

TOXICITY OF CHROMIUM

Chromium has never been shown to be toxic (in trivalent form or GTF form). The body very effectively eliminates excess amounts.[15]

SOURCES OF CHROMIUM

Brewer's yeast (not torula) is the best known source of GTF chromium. Whole grains (except rye), blackstrap molasses, black pepper, liver, cheese, sea food, meat, and nuts are also good sources.

Supplements of chromium are available. GTF chromium from brewer's yeast is preferable to inorganic chromium salts, since it is better absorbed and utilized.

19

Copper

Copper is an essential component in several enzyme systems responsible for such processes as cellular energy generation, linking of collagen, and melanin (pigment) and elastin formation. The myelin sheath which covers nerve fibers also depends on copper as a structural element. Copper catalyzes oxidation-reduction reactions, including the formation of water from hydrogen and oxygen in the body. Without copper, this reaction could be explosive. Copper is also important to the sense of taste. The utilization of iron requires copper, and copper may stimulate the absorption of iron.

A deficiency in copper causes abnormal pigmentation in the skin and hair, and defects in the elastic tissue in the blood vessels, eventually leading to rupture, anemia, faulty development of bone and nerves, and loss of the sense of taste. The only recognized occurrence of dietary copper deficiency is in infants maintained on a diet of only cow's milk for several months. (Cow's milk is a poor source of copper.) Chronic diarrhea can also cause infantile copper deficiency. Severe anemia plus osteoporosis and other bone irregularities develop in these infants.

Copper deficiency in adults is usually the result of malabsorption or extensive bowel surgery. An inherited disease, Menke's kinky hair syndrome, occurs in infants and results in slow growth, hard, twisted, kinky hair, convulsions, skeletal deformities, arterial degeneration, and progressive deterioration of the brain.[1]

Copper deficiency is quite rare. However, there is one researcher who believes it's not as rare as most scientists think. Dr. Leslie Klevay believes the American diet contains less copper than it should and that the result is cardiovascular disease.[2] Some of the effects of a copper deficiency do mimic heart disease. And recent research has shown that copper deficiency in animals raises blood levels of cholesterol.[3] However, not much additional evidence has arisen to support Dr. Klevay's hypothesis.

As a matter of fact, most research seems to center on copper's potential *toxicity*, rather than its therapeutic benefit. For example, there is a large body of evidence that copper in excess can cause mental illness. Excess copper may compete with other minerals such as zinc, manganese, and magnesium, and cause insomnia, elevated blood pressure, and restlessness. When kidney dialysis patients accumulate too much copper in their blood, they display psychotic symptoms.[4] Copper has also been found to be higher in the blood of some schizophrenics.[5]

REQUIREMENTS FOR COPPER

The RDA for copper is two to three mg. Dr. Klevay cites several studies, some of which he conducted himself, in pointing out that deficiency of copper is widespread, and that as much as eighty-four percent of the population is consuming less than the RDA. Some of the diets measured in his survey were hospital diets.[6] Another survey of military meals found that they, too, were deficient in copper.[7] None of these studies included *water* in their analysis. Many researchers feel that considerable copper enters the body through the water supply, since copper pipes are quite common, and copper dissolves in the water in great enough quantities to be a nutritional factor. Furthermore, all the diets surveyed by Dr. Klevay were institutional diets. Institutional food well deserves its reputation for mediocrity. And it's a well-known fact that the place to go to develop malnutrition is the modern hospital.

TOXICITY OF COPPER

Other than the previously mentioned references to adverse symptoms caused by copper excess, the only other report is of two blonds mysteriously becoming *greenheads* after washing their hair in water (from the tap) which had copper concentrations from thirty to sixty times normal.[8] (It is unknown whether they subsequently had more fun.)

SOURCES OF COPPER

Nuts, organ meats, seafood, mushrooms, chocolate, and legumes are the richest sources of copper. Most other fresh foods contain some copper.

Copper may be included in a multimineral supplement, or individually in small doses up to a milligram.

20

Fluorine

Of all the vitamins and minerals, fluorine is by far the most controversial. Doctors, nutritionists, and lay people will argue back and forth about the relative benefits of various vitamins and minerals. But no one joins with like-minded people marching in the streets and fighting government agencies over any of the other nutrients as people do over fluorine.

Of course, none of the other nutrients is intentionally added to public water supplies.

To many people, including most dentists, fluorine is the best thing to come along since antibiotics. To others, fluorine is a poison without redeeming qualities. Let's sort out some of the reasons why a community political firestorm erupts whenever these two groups of people find themselves looking at one another across a community fluoridation issue.

There is no definite evidence that fluorine is essential to human health. But there are studies which demonstrate that it is necessary for the growth and development of rats. On the basis of this evidence, it's reasonable to assume that humans need *trace* amounts of the mineral, too. But simply because a mineral is shown to be essential doesn't necessarily mean it can't be toxic in excess amounts. Cadmium, for example, is universally considered a poison. But the same research laboratory that established the essentiality of fluorine and of many other minerals recently found that cadmium, too, appears to be required in minute amounts.

Fluorine doesn't get into the news or the public water supply because of its essentiality in rats, however. In fact, at one time fluorine was generally considered a toxic pollutant to be especially *avoided* during the period of tooth formation in childhood! The reason for this was that teeth exposed to fluoride during their development were found to be discolored with white, yellow, or brown stains. However, government researchers also discovered that stained teeth were significantly more resistant to decay than other teeth. This led to the hypothesis that an amount of fluoride in the diet short of the amount that would cause white-yellow mottling could still help prevent tooth decay. Within ten years of these surveys and early experiments, fluoridation of public water supplies was endorsed by the United States Public Health Service.[1]

When fluorine is present during tooth development, it is incorporated into the mineral structure of the tooth. These fluorine-containing mineral crystals are supposed to be more resistant to the acids formed by the bacteria in plaque. Continued exposure of the tooth enamel to high concentrations of fluoride (from toothpaste, drinking water, or mouth rinses) is necessary to keep enamel concentrations high.[2]

TOXICITY OF FLUORINE

If the physiology of fluorine stopped there, there would be little controversy. People might have a solid argument against fluoridation of water on the grounds that it's a violation of a person's rights to add something to the water supply. This argument would probably not carry antifluoridationists too far—not because it isn't a good argument, but because there are so many things added to our water, food, and air that there is no precedent for really guarding the right to clean air, food, and water.

But there *is* a sizeable body of evidence that fluorine, or fluoride, isn't the safe, effective guardian most people, including doctors and dentists, believe it is.

The Library of Congress Research Service lists fluoride as one of the chemicals in the nation's drinking water that is increasing the risk of such diseases as cancer, heart disease, and genetic mutations. The 402-page report also said that current research and monitoring practices were unequal to the job of guarding the health of the nation.[3]

Fluoride *is* a pollutant, meaning it is a toxic waste product of industry (aluminum smelters, steel works, glass works, brick and tile works, superphosphate factories, ironstone and cryolite works, coal burning, and welding). Animals grazing close to such sources of fluoride suffer many toxic reactions to excess fluoride in their food and water. Not only do their teeth and bones become mottled, but systemic effects render them less productive.[4]

Most nutrients are essential to many enzyme reactions. Fluoride, on the other hand, is known as a potent *inhibitor* of enzymes, especially enzymes involving other metals. Fluorine's inhibition of bacterial enzymes may be how it helps protect the teeth against decay. Of course, fluoride may also inhibit important human enzyme systems.[5] In mice, fluoride (in equal concentrations to those found in fluoridated water supplies) causes chromosome damage by making the chromosomes too sticky to reproduce without damage. Chromosome damage in these mice and rats caused stillbirths, miscarriages, and birth defects.[6]

Many critics of fluoridation correctly point out that fluoride is not really as safe as other nutrients, since the difference between the amount that is supposed to help the teeth and the amount that is known to cause harm is not very great. Most fluoridated water supplies contain about 1 ppm (part per million) fluoride. In one study, between one and two percent of people using water with that concentration of fluoride had mottling covering twenty-five to fifty percent of at least two teeth. Mottling consists of paper-white opaque areas on the teeth. When the level of fluoride rose by just eighty to ninety percent to 1.8 to 1.9 ppm, brown stains began to appear. Higher concentrations have been found to result in abnormalities in the white blood cells.[7]

Of course, the concentrations of fluoride may not be as important as the *actual amount* a person takes into the body. And this is where many doctors, dentists, and public health officials apparently underestimate the danger of fluoride. A dose of .5 milligram can cause hemorrhages in the stomach and bowels, skin rash, and other serious disabilities. Doctors have found high concentrations of fluoride in body tissues of babies who have died shortly after birth, even when the mother's only source of fluoride was public water.[8] And a daily dose of 3 mg. produces mottling, whereas 5 mg. causes tooth structure to *weaken*.[9]

Many doctors and dentists believe the fatal dose level of fluoride is 2.5 to 5 grams. Actually, it's been found to be much lower. *One quarter of a milligram* can cause acute poisoning in infants. Two cases which bring home the danger of underestimating the danger of fluoride involve a public official who boasted that fluoride was eminently safe, and a three-year-old boy who was brought to the dentist for a checkup and a fluoride treatment. The public health official swallowed some fluoride tablets to show how safe they were, and landed in the hospital for more than a week. The child wasn't so lucky. He had no cavities but was given the fluoride treatment anyway. Four hours later he was dead from toxic overdose of fluoride. In the court case which followed, it was revealed that emergency room doctors let the boy wait for treatment when he could have been saved—because they underestimated the toxicity of fluoride.[10]

Some of the recognized symptoms of fluorosis—the accumulation of toxic amounts of fluoride in the body—include arthritis, muscular pain, deformities in the bones and teeth, and lesions in the gastrointestinal tract, nervous system, and eyes.[11] The primary target organs, other than the bones and teeth, of fluoride toxicity are the aorta, the thyroid, lungs, kidneys, heart, pancreas, brain, spleen, and liver.[12] The arteries store more fluoride than any other soft tissue, and many studies have reported calcification of the arteries in fluorosis.[13]

Fluorosis has also been shown to cause degeneration of the heart muscle fibers; these lesions are attributed to the blockage of vital enzyme reactions. There is evidence that this effect may also occur at chronic, lower doses. In Antigo, Wisconsin, fluoridation was temporarily halted from November, 1960, to October, 1965. Mortality from heart disease was found to be markedly higher during the periods of fluoridation. The effect seemed more pronounced among people seventy-five and over, which suggests that fluoride toxicity is related to the duration of exposure.[14]

Some people are apparently extrasensitive, or allergic, to fluoride. Doctors have reported symptoms ranging from dermatitis, acne, hives, intestinal pain, nausea, and mouth ulcers to excessive thirst, headaches, weakness, hemorrhages, and general disability. Such symptoms go away when the people no longer drink fluoridated water or stop using fluoride toothpaste.[15]

Fluoride has been used in the treatment of osteoporosis in the mistaken assumption that it help the bones retain minerals. Actually, fluoride doesn't have a normal effect on bones at all. Fluoride induces the replacement of bone with bulkier tissue which is poorly organized. Bones affected by fluoride appear denser or thicker to X-rays, but there is no evidence they are stronger.[16] Furthermore, about a quarter of the people treated with fluoride in osteoporosis suffer joint swelling, pain and gastrointestinal disorders.[17] If enough calcium is not supplied, fluoride actually causes the bones to become *demineralized*. Bone diseases such as osteomalacia and osteoporosis are high in areas where water fluoride exceeds 7 ppm.[18]

One factor many public health officials and dentists seem to be ignoring is that the total daily intake of fluoride is increasing, simply because fluoride is becoming more and more common as a *pollutant*. Fluoride in air pollution has been severe enough to cause several deaths during air inversions.[19] The lesson many researchers seem to be learning from studies of widespread toxicity of fluoride is that the *sum* of all exposures to fluoride must be accounted for, not just the concentrations in drinking water. And they are learning that this total is increasing.[20] For example, one doctor reported that foods such as infant formulas, processed infant food, and dry milk mixed with fluoridated water can sometimes result in fluoride concentrations of from 4 to 12 ppm.[21]

Several countries have outlawed fluoridation, including France, Italy, Denmark, and Norway. In West Germany, Belgium, and Japan, the governments discourage further fluoridation. Sweden has repealed fluoridation. Holland only allows it where an alternative water supply is present. In Britain, Canada, and the United States, the controversy rages on.

21

Iodine

Iodine has one recognized role in human health, and that is in the formation of thyroxin, the thyroid hormone. Thyroxin regulates the metabolic rate of the body, and the availability of iodine affects the amount of hormone secreted. When there is a deficiency of iodine, the thyroid attempts to compensate by secreting more thyroxin. The gland then becomes enlarged, swollen, and congested. This is known as *goiter*. If insufficient iodine is present in a developing fetus, physical and mental retardation—cretinism—can result.

Goiter and cretinism are known to occur in areas of the world where iodine is low or nonexistent in the food supply. In some countries, such as the United States, iodine deficiency goiter (endemic goiter) has been virtually wiped out by fortifying table salt with *iodide*. Iodine deficiency, however, still affects upwards of 200 million people around the world.[1]

Iodine is controversial for two reasons. The first is because an American researcher has performed epidemiological studies and found that breast, uterine, and ovarian cancer seem to be lower in areas of the world where iodine intake is high. Low intake of iodine may stimulate production of hormones which could help cause these forms of cancer.[2] Keep in mind that this is only a theory based on studies of cancer death rates and iodine intake. Other factors obviously enter into the causation of cancer, and further experimentation is required before this theory is adequately tested.

Iodine is controversial, too, because many researchers now consider it a pollutant rather than a necessary supplement. They maintain that not only is iodine plentiful enough in the environment to stop putting it in salt, but that perhaps it's too plentiful for our own good.

The RDA for iodine is 150 micrograms (.15 mg.). Two grams of iodized salt supplies at least this amount. However, Americans consume, on the average, five times that much salt every day. And several other factors have raised the average daily exposure to iodine even further. Dairy cows are exposed to high concentrations of iodine in iodized salt blocks, iodine-containing disinfectants, and supplemented feed. Iodine may reach levels as high as 450 micrograms per quart of milk. Bakeries use iodine compounds as dough conditioners. Erythrosine, a red food dye, also contributes significant quantities of iodine. Many drugs contain iodine. And burning fossil fuels and organic matter also results in iodine air pollution.[3] Nuclear power plants leak substantial amounts of deadly, cancer-causing radioactive iodine. Studies have shown that areas within thirty miles of a plant can experience a doubling of the thyroid cancer rate.[4]

Thyroid toxicity (thyrotoxicosis) has been reported to occur after administration of iodine supplements. Apparently, an excess of iodine results in the same physiological effect as a deficiency: hyperthyroidism. Many people react adversely to levels of iodine which are safe for most others, suggesting they have some metabolic defect which interferes with the regulation of the iodine-thyroid system.[5] In addition to the stepped-up metabolism of hyperthyroidism and thyrotoxicosis, an excess of iodine can also cause acne.[6]

Several studies, including the Ten State Nutrition Survey, have found that people in the United States with goiter do not have it because of a deficiency of iodine. These people generally excrete not only many times the amount of iodine used as a cutoff point to indicate a deficiency, but they also excrete more than the people who don't have goiter.[7] This suggests that these people may have defects in their iodine-thyroid regulation.

The best natural sources of iodine are seafoods, including fish *and* seaweeds. A diet with plenty of these items does not need iodine supplementation. Baked goods and milk may also provide iodine, although it is not a natural part of the food, and is not a reliable source. Your baker may not use iodine compounds as dough conditioners; your dairy may not use iodine salt licks and disinfectants. Iodine is still an essential mineral. The best way to make sure you're getting enough, without increasing your salt intake, is to eat seafood.

22

Iron

Long before vitamin and mineral supplements were any more than a rather cultish practice enjoyed by "faddists" in California and a few big cities, millions of people took iron supplements every day. They did so because television, radio, and print advertising told them they should do so to avoid "tired blood."

Surprisingly, the TV commercials were right. A lot of people do have "tired" blood—blood which does not carry enough oxygen to the cells to keep bodily functions operating at optimum efficiency. And many people do need to take iron supplements to correct this deficiency.

WHAT IRON DOES

Iron is the primary component of hemoglobin, which is the part of the red blood cell that carries oxygen from the lungs to the cells and carbon dioxide from the cells to the lungs. Iron is also an essential component of myoglobin, which is a receptor and storage point for some of the oxygen in the muscles. Iron is also essential to the intracellular cytochrome system, which is another part of energy production.

An adult's body contains from 3 to 5 grams of iron. About 1 gram of this is stored in the liver. When red blood cells are broken down at the end of their useful life, their iron content is salvaged fairly efficiently in most people. Nevertheless, iron losses still occur in sweat, hair, lost skin, bleeding, and excretion. A normal adult male loses about 1 mg. of iron a day, while a woman can lose from 1 to 2 mg. During menstruation, injury, and bleeding, significantly higher quantities are lost.

WHAT HAPPENS WHEN IRON DEMAND EXCEEDS SUPPLY

Since iron is needed by all the cells of the body, and since every cell depends on oxygen, a deficiency of iron can have widespread effects. Anemia is a result of iron deficiency: the amount of circulating hemoglobin is markedly diminished. The red blood cells become pale, and cannot deliver as much oxygen to the cells as may be needed. The general symptoms are pallor, weakness, easy fatigability, labored breathing on exertion, headache, palpitation, and persistent tiredness. Iron deficiency sometimes results in a form of pica (perverted appetite for an item not usually considered food). In this case, the appetite is for *ice* (pagophagia).[1] Dry scaling of the lips, spoon nails, and hair fall can also occur.[2]

Iron deficiency anemia has been found to depress the immune system. White blood cells are reduced in their bacteria-killing activity. In two groups of children with anemia and depressed immunity, iron supplements greatly improved their ability to fight off infections.[3] Iron deficiency has been shown to enhance the growth of tumors induced in animals by chemicals or viruses.[4] Iron deficiency also causes degeneration of the periodontal tissue in animals.[5]

As might be expected, an iron deficiency will reduce the body's capacity for work. In one study, performance on a treadmill was found to be proportional to the hemoglobin levels in the blood of seventy-five women between the ages of twenty-two and sixty-five.[6] In a Swedish study, oral iron supplements (120 mg. per day) were found to increase work capacity about four percent in men and twelve percent in women between the ages of fifty-eight and seventy-one.[7]

Preschool children have been found to suffer diminished coordination, balance, attention span, intelligence quotient, and memory when anemic. Iron supplements have succeeded in restoring normal function.[8] In older children, anemia has been shown to cause poorer learning, reading, and problem-solving skills.[9]

In animal experiments, a deficiency of iron has been shown to increase both the absorption and toxicity of lead.[10] Conversely, lead absorption and toxicity can be diminished or prevented by iron in the diet.[11]

Iron in excess of nutritional requirements has also been shown to completely prevent the toxicity of cadmium in animals. Vitamin C's protection against cadmium toxicity has been shown to rely heavily on the vitamin's ability to increase the amount of iron that is absorbed and made available to the cells.[12]

REQUIREMENTS FOR IRON

The RDA for iron is 10 to 15 mg. for infants, 15 to 20 mg. for children, 10 to 18 mg. for adolescents and adults, and 18 mg. for pregnant and lactating women. These figures are based on estimates of how much iron must be ingested to make up for average daily losses. (Normal daily losses are about 1 to 2 mg.) But not all the iron in the diet is absorbed. Nutrition scientists believe less than ten percent is absorbed, so to make up for losses of 2 mg., more than 20 mg. must be supplied in the diet. Of course, many factors can raise requirements, including pregnancy, blood loss, and injury. During the entire course of a pregnancy, for example, the fetus requires a total of from 300 to 500 mg. of iron for development. This is in addition to the mother's own needs. Supplements as high as 60 mg. per day, however, have been found to be inadequate to raise hemoglobin levels to normal in some pregnant women.[13]

Just *how many* people are actually deficient in iron is one of the great nutrition controversies of our time—not because it's especially *heated*, as in the fluoride controversy, but because the range of opinions is so broad. Depending on whose study you read and whose figures you decide to believe, between two percent and ninety-five percent of a given population is deficient in iron. Because iron status is usually measured according to hemoglobin count, and because hemoglobin counts are quite variable, whether a person is judged anemic depends on what level of hemoglobin the doctor decides is normal. The Food and Drug Administration, usually quite conservative when it comes to recommending supplements, has reported that most pregnant women, adolescent girls, menstruating women, and infants are not receiving adequate iron in their diets.

And the Food and Nutrition Board, also not given to recommending supplements, has also acknowledged that the typical American diet cannot supply enough iron to meet the RDA of 18 mg.[14]

Meals from fifty colleges were found to be consistently deficient in iron.[15] A relatively small sampling of college women found that twenty-four percent were deficient in iron. And the Ten State Nutrition Survey found that twenty-two percent of adult *males* were deficient in iron.[16] Another group in jeopardy for iron deficiency is formula-fed infants. Even infants receiving formulas *fortified* with iron have lower hemoglobin levels than breastfed infants.[17]

There is disagreement over whether iron absorption increases during a deficiency. Some sources say that a deficiency *does* increase the efficiency of iron in food and supplements, while others say only supplemental iron is absorbed more efficiently in a deficiency. The duodenum (first section of the small intestine) is the site of iron absorption. The mucous membrane of the intestine prevents an overload of iron in the body by absorbing iron less efficiently when stores are high. It's reasonable to assume this regulation can extend to absorbing more iron when stores are low.

Many other factors can affect the absorption and utilization of iron. Any condition that includes loss of blood, of course, raises iron requirements. Iron is poorly absorbed in the presence of phosphates, oxalates and phytates (common substances in foods). Egg yolks impair iron absorption. Iron from animal sources is absorbed better than iron from plants, and absorption of iron from plants is enhanced in the presence of meat. Iron is also absorbed better in the presence of acids. Vitamin C, ascorbic acid, can boost iron absorption as much as tenfold when ingested at the same meal. A fairly common food additive used as a preservative, EDTA (ethylenediaminetetraacetate), is a powerful anti-iron absorption agent. Amounts of EDTA equal to those possible in an American diet have been shown to reduce iron absorption to one-fifth of normal. EDTA even negates the iron absorption-enhancing effect of vitamin C.[18]

TOXICITY OF IRON

Because the body regulates the amount of iron absorbed, it is not normally possible to produce toxicity from dietary or supplemental iron, since any excess is simply excreted. However, there is an inherited disorder of iron-absorption regulation, *hemochromatosis*, which allows toxic levels of iron to be absorbed. In a Swedish study of 347 people, four men were found with early biochemical signs of hemochromatosis. No women were found with iron overload.[19]

SOURCES OF IRON

Natural sources of iron include liver, heart, kidney, lean

meats, shellfish, dried beans and fruits, nuts, green leafy vegetables, whole grains, and blackstrap molasses. Some studies have found that the iron used to fortify processed cereals is poorly absorbed.[20] Iron in mother's milk is five times more efficiently absorbed than iron in cow's milk or formula. Assuming a nursing mother has sufficient iron stores, a breastfed infant does not need iron supplements.[21]

Iron supplements are available in a wide range of doses, from 1 mg. to 60 mg. or more, and a wide variety of forms: ferrous sulphate, ferrous gluconate, ferrous fumarate, etc. Iron is also available in syrup form, sometimes mixed with vitamins.

23

Magnesium

We tend to take magnesium for granted. Most people probably don't even know it's an essential mineral. Our body can't forget about magnesium, however, because the mineral plays *the* central role in regulating cell metabolism and growth. Almost all the chemical reactions the cell must carry out depend on magnesium.[1]

On a less fundamental level, magnesium is essential for the activation of several important enzyme reactions, including those that transfer phosphate from adenosine triphosphate (ATP) to adenosine diphosphate (ADP). ATP-ADP reactions are basic to all life processes.

Cardiac and skeletal muscles must have a correct balance of calcium and magnesium in order to function properly. Nerve transmission also depends on the balance between calcium and magnesium in the blood.

WHAT HAPPENS WHEN MAGNESIUM DEMAND EXCEEDS SUPPLY

Low levels of magnesium in body fluids increase nerve conduction, and by stepping up the transmission of nerve impulses, these low levels increase muscular irritability and contractibility. In a severe deficiency, muscle tremors, uncontrolled movements of the hands and the face, and convulsions can occur.

Magnesium deficiency can result in an imbalance in calcium metabolism, with the mineral being deposited in the soft tissues. Bone deformities also occur. Magnesium deficiency also leads to degeneration of the kidneys, skeletal and cardiac muscle, endocardium, skin, and teeth. Blood levels of calcium and potassium are depressed. Sodium accumulates in the tissues, and edema results.[2] And remember, local tissue deficiencies of magnesium can occur without blood levels falling below normal.[3]

In animals, magnesium deficiency diminishes the ability to adapt to cold. Deficient animals suffer ulceration, calcification of the kidney, heart and blood vessels, damage to the heart, and reduced lifespan.[4] In some experiments, magnesium deficiency caused seizures and a reduced motivation to learn in rats. When the animals were forced to perform in order to survive, they did. But voluntary activity was markedly impaired.[5]

In humans, magnesium deficiency can cause a wide variety of symptoms, including lethargy, muscular weakness, knotting of muscle and nerve fibers (fasciculation), gross tremors, tetany, writing movements of the hands, irritability, mental changes, convulsions, stupor, coma, dizziness, psychotic behavior, exaggeration of the reflexes, jerks, and seizures.[6] In babies and children, magnesium deficiency can cause loss of appetite, growth failure, apathy, irritability, hallucinations, confusion, weakness, flaccidity, occasional spasticity and rigidity, tremors, twitches, apnea (breathing stops), and rapid pulse. Some researchers believe there may be a connection between magnesium deficiency and sudden infant death syndrome.[7]

Neonatal tetany (convulsions) often results from a magnesium deficiency, even though the major biochemical sign is low calcium levels in the blood. These infants will often respond to magnesium supplementation (injected) better than to calcium, presumably because the magnesium deficiency is causing the severe drop in blood levels of calcium.[8] And magnesium can be crucial to calcium metabolism; rickets will sometimes respond to magnesium supplementation after massive doses of vitamin D have failed.[9]

Magnesium and Heart Disease

Recent evidence has led many doctors to suggest that dietary magnesium may be a preventive factor in heart disease. Beginning with evidence from animal experiments, a low-magnesium diet produces structural and functional degeneration of the heart in rats. In a study of human hearts, heart muscle tissue from heart attack victims had markedly less magnesium than tissue from the hearts of people without heart disease. Areas of the heart that were undersupplied with oxygen (but not totally deprived) also were lower than normal tissue in magnesium.

Doctors believe these local tissue deficiencies in the heart may predispose such hearts to fatal arrhythmias, or make them more vulnerable to damage during oxygen deprivation (infarct).[10] Since magnesium turnover occurs at a more rapid rate in the heart than in any other tissue, the heart is affected by a deficiency before other tissues. This damage may not become apparent until it is too late.[11] Magnesium levels in the hearts of men dying from heart attack have been found to be much lower than in hearts of men dying from other causes.[12] And heart attack victims who survive, as well as people with coronary insufficiency, have also been found to have lower-than-normal blood levels of magnesium. In most, these low levels return to normal slowly after about twelve days from the time of the attack.[13]

Several studies around the world have established that heart disease death rates are higher in areas where the water is soft than where the water is hard. Attempts to determine what factor in the hard water seems to contribute to the difference have come up with many factors, one of which is magnesium. Heart tissue concentrations of all minerals *except magnesium* are about the same in many hard-water and soft-water areas. Recent epidemiological work has found that magnesium apparently lowers the rate of "sudden deaths" from cardiac arrhythmias (severe disturbance of the heart's normal rhythm).[14]

Since a magnesium deficiency results in increased muscular excitability, it's not difficult to understand how a deficiency in the heart muscle could cause the heart to spasm and lose its normal rhythm. As a matter of fact, a study in which magnesium supplements were given to twenty heart patients found that the mineral *did* decrease the risk of ventricular fibrillation (a sudden twitching of the heart that halts the pumping of blood).[15] Actually, over the years many doctors have used magnesium to *treat* cardiac arrhythmias of both spontaneous origin and those caused by the drug digitalis.[16]

Doctors have reported magnesium to be of use in the treatment of people with ischemic heart disease, that the mineral may increase survival and relieve pain after a heart attack. It is also not unreasonable to assume that magnesium can *help prevent* heart disease, too. Foods that are usually associated with increased risk of heart disease—fats, refined carbohydrates and sugars, and alcoholic beverages—are also quite low in magnesium. Fruits, vegetables, lean meats, fish, and legumes, all beneficial foods, happen to be high in magnesium. While no one would presume that magnesium is the sole factor in preventing heart disease, the mineral is undeniably very important, and arranging your diet to avoid low-magnesium foods in favor of high-magnesium foods will contribute to avoiding heart attack.[17]

Magnesium and "Housewife Syndrome"

The doctor who reported magnesium's use in "housewife syndrome" describes the malady as "fatigue in the morning after what should have been an adequate night's sleep, and a lassitude that, although less severe in the morning, rapidly increases during the day, with utter exhaustion by nightfall." Added to these are vague pains, tension headaches, insomnia despite tiredness, and lower back pain. Of course, these symptoms could be found in *anyone* with a full day of work ahead of them.

Nevertheless, the doctor used supplements of magnesium and potassium, and succeeded in alleviating many of the symptoms in eighty-seven percent of the women *(and men)* treated. The subjects became aware of an increase in energy and strength, and almost all undertook new activities, including part-time jobs outside the home.[18]

Magnesium is also used successfully by many doctors to control high blood pressure in women with eclampsia of pregnancy. Magnesium also controls the convulsions of eclampsia, which threaten the baby during labor, and the mineral is not only safer but more effective than other agents.[19]

Magnesium supplements have also been used by many doctors to treat nervousness, insomnia (sometimes with calcium), and muscle cramps and spasms.[20]

REQUIREMENTS FOR MAGNESIUM

The RDA for magnesium ranges from 60 mg. for infants up to 450 mg. for pregnant or lactating women. For adult men it is 350 mg.; for adult women, 300 mg. These figures are not based on any evidence of *need*, but rather are figured from estimates of how much the typical American diet *provides*. This doesn't seem like a very reliable way to determine nutrient requirements, unless you're considering the convenience of the food processors.

As a matter of fact, the Western diet supplies only *suboptimal* amounts of magnesium. Males are especially susceptible to a dietary deficiency.[21] One reason for this is that women are apparently better able to metabolize magnesium than men.[22] Although the body absorbs magnesium more efficiently in a deficiency, normal absorption of the mineral is slow and incomplete (only about ten percent is absorbed). Absorption may be reduced by fat, phytates (phosphorus compounds in some foods, which can diminish intestinal absorption of minerals), and calcium. General protein-calorie malnutrition also reduces the absorption of magnesium.

Many circumstances can raise metabolic requirements for magnesium, including trauma, burns, wounds, and dietary calcium, phosphorus, and protein.[23] Magnesium deficiency occurs in many conditions and diseases, including congestive heart failure, diabetes, alcoholism, cirrhosis, malabsorption syndromes, after surgery, pancreatitis, endocrine disorders, renal disease, and prolonged diarrhea.[24] Magnesium has also been found low in people treated with antidepressant drugs.[25]

TOXICITY OF MAGNESIUM

Excess magnesium taken orally has a laxative effect. People have been taking advantage of this for many generations by using epsom salts.

If blood levels of magnesium get extremely high, the depressing effect on neuromuscular irritability may produce lethargy, loss of reflexes, anesthesia, and drowsiness. Since the intestines regulate magnesium absorption, and allow less of the mineral into the bloodstream when blood levels are already adequate, it is unlikely that normal supplemental doses would come anywhere near causing these effects. These effects have been reported when doctors have administered high doses of magnesium directly into the bloodstream.[26]

SOURCES OF MAGNESIUM

Natural foods all contain some magnesium. Rich sources include legumes, nuts, and whole grains. Meats are relatively poor sources, although shellfish are high in magnesium. Magnesium is removed from grains and many other foods when they are refined, so white flour is a poor source of magnesium, as are other refined grains.[27] College meals are apparently not a good source of magnesium, since one study of meals from fifty colleges found them consistently deficient in magnesium.[28]

Magnesium is also available in supplement form, usually as magnesium oxide, in doses ranging from 50 to 500 mg.

24

Manganese

Manganese is one of the most common elements in the earth's crust. All animal and plant tissues, as well as all fresh and sea water, rain water, and atmospheric dust, contain manganese. Human tissue has not yet been found that doesn't contain some manganese. Manganese is considered an essential trace mineral because it is an essential cofactor in several vital enzyme systems. Manganese functions in the synthesis of protein, DNA and RNA, and cartilage.[1] Manganese also plays a role in the utilization of insulin, and it may be essential to metabolism of fats as well. There are reports of a preparation of alfalfa, high in manganese, being used in African folk medicine as a treatment for diabetes.[2]

A deficiency of manganese causes impairment of growth, reproduction, glucose tolerance, egg shell formation, blood clotting, and skeletal deformities and loss of muscular coordination.[3] Manganese deficiency has also been found to lower the immune response in animals.[4] Manganese deficiency has been found to be responsible for certain birth defects in animals, once thought to be caused by genetic mutations. Supplying manganese supplements to pregnant animals erased the effects in offspring.[5]

In humans, the symptoms of a manganese deficiency were discovered by accident when manganese was mistakenly left out of a test diet. The volunteer experienced weight loss, dermatitis, nausea, slow growth of hair and beard with color changes, and uncommonly low blood levels of cholesterol.[6]

In a study comparing trace mineral levels in the diet with death rates from cardiovascular disease, manganese was one of the minerals (along with chromium and selenium) that were found to be high in areas where heart-disease deaths were low, and low where heart-disease deaths were high.[7]

South African doctors made use of that folk remedy—alfalfa—and successfully controlled the blood sugar of a young diabetic who was not responding to insulin. They reported that the alfalfa was very high in manganese, and that the mineral was responsible for lowering blood sugar by potentiating the action of insulin.[8]

Canadian doctors discovered a link between manganese levels and epileptic seizures. While routinely checking for lead poisoning in a child with epilepsy, they found extremely low levels of manganese. They then checked the blood of the other children in the Convulsive Disorders Clinic, and found that one-third of the children had lower manganese levels than normal children. Manganese supplements were given to the first child, and his condition improved: fewer seizures, and better speech, learning, and gait. Because manganese deficiency in pregnant animals produces offspring with convulsive disorders, the doctors believe manganese deficiency during human pregnancy may be a factor in epilepsy.[9]

Schizophrenia patients, especially those with tardive dyskinesia (see Choline chapter) have been found to have abnormally low blood levels of manganese. Manganese supplementation (15 to 60 mg. per day) was found to either prevent or alleviate tardive dyskinesia in most people suffering this side effect of psychiatric drugs.[10]

Manganese toxicity has been reported in miners breathing high-manganese dust for extended periods of time. The symptoms were identical to Parkinsonism. The manganese was absorbed through the lungs, and not the digestive tract. High dietary levels are toxic in animals, however.[11]

Although manganese is known to be essential, no RDA has been determined. There is no extensive research involving manganese status in the general population, other than that described.

The best natural sources of manganese include whole grains, wheat germ and bran, peas, tea, ginger, and sage. Wine, nuts, leafy vegetables, and fruits are fair sources.

Manganese is sometimes included in multimineral supplements.

25

Molybdenum

Molybdenum is a relatively rare mineral, yet it appears to be essential, since it shows up in minute concentrations in all plant and animal tissues. Molybdenum is known to be a cofactor in some important enzyme systems, such as those involved in energy production, urine formation, and fatty acid oxidation. The mineral is necessary for plant growth, and has been used to boost crops and livestock production in areas where it is deficient in the soil.[1]

The only reports involving molybdenum and humans concern possible stimulation of hemoglobin synthesis when used with iron therapy in anemia.[2] There are no reports of molybdenum deficiency, although such a deficiency is theoretically possible because refining of grains and sugars removes most of the molybdenum.[3] Major sources of the mineral are legumes, organ meats, and milk. Multimineral tablets may contain small amounts of molybdenum, but it is not a common supplement.

Molybdenum is toxic in excess amounts. All toxicity reports have involved animals, however.

26

Phosphorus

Phosphorus may have more functions than any other mineral in the body. Nevertheless, because it is so common in the environment and the food supply, there is more concern over getting *too much* of it than over not getting enough.

Phosphorus teams with calcium to give bones and teeth their rigidity. Skeletal tissue contains about eighty percent of the body's phosphorus. The rest resides in body fluids and in every cell in the body. *Every* metabolic process in the body requires phosphorus, including muscle energy production, carbohydrate, fat, and protein metabolism, blood chemistry, nervous tissue metabolism, fatty acid transport, and numerous enzyme systems.

A phosphorus deficiency would cause demineralization of the bones or defective formation of the bones in children. Because vitamin D regulates the absorption of phosphorus, as it does calcium, a deficiency of vitamin D could cause a deficiency in phosphorus, too. Phosphorus deficiency is also possible in several disease states, including alcoholism, malabsorption, diabetic ketoacidosis, sepsis, renal defects, hyperthyroidism, osteoporosis of disuse, and hyperparathyroidism. Intravenous glucose therapy and antacids can also cause phosphorus depletion.[1]

Most of the controversy surrounding phosphorus involves its potential toxicity. Several studies have attempted to determine the exact effect of excess phosphorus on calcium balance and bone mineralization. Excess levels of phosphorus in the blood depress calcium levels low enough to stimulate parathyroid hormone secretion, which causes resorption of bone to increase. Apparently, excess phosphorus lowers calcium levels by "flushing" the mineral out of the blood.[2] In rats, a high-phosphorus diet lowers blood levels of calcium and increases bone mineral loss.[3] In people, excess phosphorus has the same effect: calcium blood levels drop and calcium levels in the feces rise, indicating that calcium is being mobilized from bones and eliminated from the body.[4]

Most concern about the high levels of phosphorus in our diet is directed at processed food. Phosphate additives show up in more and more processed food every day, despite research which has demonstrated that these phosphates are even more dangerous to the health of our bones and teeth than naturally occurring phosphorus.

In one study, volunteers were fed a diet containing no phosphate additives for four weeks, then given foods off the supermarket shelves with phosphate additives. With little or no change in the types of foods, and with no change in the total calories ingested, the switch to processed foods more than *doubled* the volunteers' phosphorus intake. This was immediately accompanied by intestinal distress, soft stools, and mild diarrhea. Even though the diet contained slightly more calcium, blood levels of calcium dropped, and phosphorus rose; and though urinary levels of calcium dropped, fecal levels rose significantly, indicating that calcium was being taken from the bones and excreted. The researchers concluded that a diet of commercially available processed foods may contain more than two and a half times the RDA for phosphorus (800 mg. for adults), and that a calcium-phosphorus ratio similar to that which resulted in calcium loss (1:2.8) could easily occur.[5]

Other researchers found that the phosphorus compounds (phosphates) used as food additives were *more likely* than naturally occurring phosphorus to cause calcium imbalance and loss, because they have a greater affinity for calcium and will combine with it more readily.[6]

Natural sources of phosphorus include meat, fish, poultry, eggs, milk, cheese, nuts, and legumes. Phosphorus is sometimes found in multimineral or calcium supplements, primarily because it frequently occurs with calcium in natural sources used in supplements.

27

Potassium

Potassium is one of the most abundant minerals in the human body. A 150-pound person has about 250 grams (nine ounces) of potassium in his or her body. Many cellular enzyme systems depend on potassium, and nerve excitation and muscular contraction are influenced by the mineral.

A deficiency in potassium can cause muscular weakness, increased nervous irritability, mental disorientation, and cardiac irregularities. If blood levels of potassium get low enough, ventricular fibrillation (in which the heart vibrates rather than pumps) can occur and cause sudden death.[1] Muscle weakness, deterioration, and periodic paralysis from potassium deficiency are quite common.[2]

Potassium and Sodium-Induced High Blood Pressure

Excess sodium in the diet can cause high blood pressure.[3] Less publicized, however, is the equally well-established ability of potassium to counteract the effect of sodium in raising blood pressure. In animal experiments, potassium added to the diets of rats fed excess sodium not only extended lifespan but reduced blood pressure raised by the sodium. (Some experiments with rats have not demonstrated the lowering of blood pressure, but lifespan was still extended by potassium. But in these experiments, the amount of excess sodium fed the animals was only moderate, and the rise in blood pressure was slight.)[4]

Human experiments have also shown that potassium can protect against the blood pressure-raising effect of a high-sodium diet. Some experiments have demonstrated that sodium salts cause a rise in blood pressure while potassium salts cause a decline. And some have shown that potassium can keep blood pressure low *despite* high sodium levels in the diet. These effects are not universal, however. Not all hypertension is from excess sodium intake. Some doctors believe that some people (especially blacks) may be more susceptible than others to the effects of sodium, that just about *everybody* is vulnerable to some extent, and that potassium can offer some protection.[5]

One recent study has found that the amount of potassium in the diet was a more important cause of high blood pressure than was the amount of sodium. High dietary levels of sodium resulted in high blood pressure only when potassium levels were low. And *low* sodium levels in the diet were also found to result in high blood pressure, if potassium levels were also low.[6]

Potassium is related to the problem of cardiovascular disease in another way. Studies have shown that people dying suddenly from heart attack (myocardial infarction) have low levels of potassium in the heart tissue.[7]

Do these reports mean that taking potassium supplements will lower your blood pressure and reduce your risk of dying of cardiovascular disease? No research has been done to answer that question directly. The evidence suggests that potassium *can* protect against the toxic effect of sodium. Doctors also know that reducing the amount of sodium in the diet will also lower blood pressure in many people. But again, the beneficial or protective effect of a single nutrient should not be taken as "the answer" to anything. Do not expect potassium supplements to protect you completely from the harmful effects of excess salt consumption, lack of exercise, fatty diet, and stressful lifestyle.

Potassium and "Housewife Syndrome"

(See Magnesium Chapter)

REQUIREMENTS FOR POTASSIUM

There is no established RDA for potassium, but authorities recommend that potassium intake should equal sodium intake, or about 2.6 grams per day. The National Research Council suggests that a daily intake between 1.87 grams and 5.6 grams should be "safe and adequate."

Potassium requirements can be raised by many factors besides sodium intake, including vomiting, gastric drainage, alcoholism, renal disease, and anorexia. Drugs which can cause a potassium deficiency include purgatives, laxatives, ammonium chloride, corticosteroids, carbenoxolone, carbenicillin, aminosalicylic acid, amphoterin, diuretics, glucagon, insulin, penicillin, and silver nitrate. Licorice eaten in excess has produced severe drops in potassium levels in the blood.[8] Acute stress, trauma, or surgery can also cause a sudden deficit in potassium, with resultant impairment of glucose tolerance.[9]

Probably the most common factor affecting potassium requirements is exercise or work. Substantial portions of the body's potassium can be lost in sweat. In human experiments, volunteers lost more than half their total body potassium after running eighteen to twenty miles in warm, humid weather. Diets with the recommended levels of potassium (2.6 grams) were adequate to replace potassium lost in the urine and feces, but not to replace that which was lost in sweat, and that amounted to more than what was lost through the other channels. These studies have shown that athletes who sweat profusely—and, presumably, nonathletes who also work up a sweat—might need anywhere from 3 to 6 grams of potassium a day.[10] If potassium depletion continues, destruction of the muscle tissue can result.[11]

TOXICITY OF POTASSIUM

Potassium can be toxic in excess. When buying supplements, avoid enteric-coated, time-release tablets, since these can cause dangerous small-bowel perforations.[12] Acute toxicity occurs with daily doses of as little as 25 grams of potassium chloride per day. Smaller doses may cause diarrhea.[13] Potassium excess can cause cardiac arrhythmia, weakness, anxiety, low blood pressure, confusion, and loss of sensation in the extremities.[14]

SOURCES OF POTASSIUM

Natural food sources of potassium include bananas, lettuce, broccoli, potatoes, fresh fruit, peanuts (unsalted!), wheat germ, squash, nuts, and orange juice.

Potassium is removed from many processed foods. In fact, many of the same processing steps that remove potassium also add sodium. Food processors add salt to foods to "enhance" flavor. Many doctors believe salt is addictive, in the sense that we grow accustomed to the salty taste of foods and learn to "need" salt on just about everything. Food processors start us off on the "habit" at birth with infant formulas containing salt, and continue it with baby foods loaded with salt.

One source of potassium that acknowledges our need for salt is the potassium salt substitute. Actually, there are cultures in the world that avoid sodium salt like the plague, and use *only* potassium salt. Several of these substitutes are available.

Potassium is also available in supplementary form in a wide range of doses. Potassium salts are among the most heavily prescribed drugs.[15]

28

Selenium

For many years, selenium was considered a poison. But for the last two decades, evidence of its essential role in human health has steadily accumulated. Now, not only is it recognized as a required nutrient, but recent research reveals that it plays a very important role in fighting two of the most ominous threats to optimum health: cancer and heart disease.

Selenium plays important or essential roles in many functions, including antioxidation, several enzyme systems, maintenance of the integrity of muscle cells and red blood cells, DNA-RNA synthesis, detoxification of poisonous metals, cellular respiration and energy transfer, production of sperm cells, fetal development, integrity of keratinous tissue (skin, hair, nails), pancreatic function, antibody synthesis, and the production of *ubiquinones* (substances believed to help protect against infectious diseases and malignancies, inflammatory diseases, heart disease, and high blood pressure).[1]

Selenium's role as an antioxidant has received much attention in research, because oxidative damage to cells and cell membranes is known to occur in most diseases and in aging. It was once thought that selenium might act as an antioxidant by actually combining with oxygen itself, much the same way vitamin E protects cells and membranes. However, recent research has discovered that selenium instead is an essential component of *glutathione peroxidase*, an enzyme which destroys *hydroperoxide*, a very potent oxidizer.

Glutathione peroxidase has been found to be involved in resistance to several disease states. Low levels of the enzyme are found in drug treatments, neonatal jaundice, alcoholic liver disease, and blood clotting disorders. Glutathione protects cells from oxidation and mutation by various substances. It's involved in carbohydrate metabolism and prostaglandin metabolism. White blood cells and red blood cells also depend on glutathione peroxidase for proper function. Peroxidation of fats is known to be involved in cardiovascular disease, and glutathione peroxidase is known to break down peroxides in the fats.[2]

Selenium's role in glutathione peroxidase synthesis is also important because it helps explain the apparent "teamwork" between selenium and vitamin E. This teamwork was discovered when animals thought to be suffering from vitamin E deficiencies were given supplements of the vitamin—to no avail. Selenium was subsequently identified as the missing factor, and later experiments further documented that selenium deficiency could cause many of the symptoms of oxidative damage in a vitamin E deficit.[3]

Selenium can also *prevent* some of the damage which occurs when there is a vitamin E deficiency.[4]

WHAT HAPPENS WHEN SELENIUM DEMAND EXCEEDS SUPPLY?

Because selenium is involved in so many important biological processes, and because the mineral is not uniformly distributed, it's no surprise that some forty animal species are known to suffer disorders attributed to selenium deficiency. Animal feeds are routinely supplemented with selenium in order to prevent these diseases. Animals deficient in selenium show calcification and degeneration of the muscle and lesions in the blood vessels of the heart. Liver tissue loses its ability to take up oxygen and dies. The integrity of the cell membrane is severely compromised and the membrane becomes "leaky." Fluid which leaks from the cells and membranes collects, and intracellular enzymes leak into the blood.[5] Selenium deficiency causes infertility in males, by causing testicular degeneration with severe impairment of sperm motility as the first manifestation. In females, selenium deficiency causes infertility by fetal death and resorption.[6]

In a selenium deficiency, vitamin E metabolism increases and may result in an increased requirement for the vitamin.[7] Selenium deficiency also enhances the damaging effects of ozone on the lungs.[8] And since premature infants are lower in selenium than normal-term infants, selenium deficiency has been implicated in oxidative damage to the lungs and eyes of premature infants given oxygen therapy.[9]

A selenium deficiency, of course, also results in a deficiency of glutathione peroxidase. At one time, this enzyme deficiency was thought to be exclusively hereditary.[10]

Selenium and Heart Disease

Since a selenium deficiency affects the functional and structural integrity of the cardiovascular system in animals, researchers suspect it may play a role in human heart disease. Comparisons of selenium bioavailability and intake with death rates for heart disease have turned up some very interesting statistics. In areas of the world where selenium is high (over twenty-five countries have been studied), death rates for cardiovascular, renal, cerebrovascular, coronary and hypertensive heart disease tend to be significantly lower. Cities with high selenium intake have death rates for arteriosclerotic and hypertensive heart disease which are lower than the expected rate according to national statistics.[11]

A combination of selenium (500 micrograms) and vitamin E (100 IU) was tested on heart patients with angina. Out of twenty-four people given the supplements, twenty-two experienced a significant reduction in angina pain. Only five out of twenty-four people reported any benefit when a placebo tablet was given to them instead of the vitamin-mineral supplement.[12]

Selenium and Cancer

Selenium was once thought to be carcinogenic, but scientists now know that even in doses that *are* toxic, selenium does not cause cancer. In fact, evidence seems to point in the other direction, that selenium helps *protect against* cancer. As with heart disease, epidemiological evidence from the United States and several other countries demonstrates that where selenium levels are high, cancer death rates tend to be lower than where selenium is not as available. Researchers have broken down the data and found that certain types of cancer are more "responsive" to selenium variations. These include cancers of the tongue, esophagus, stomach, intestine, rectum, liver, pancreas, larynx, lung, kidney, prostate, bladder, lymph glands, breast, thyroid, and uterus.[13]

A somewhat closer relationship between selenium and cancer has been found in that blood levels of selenium in cancer patients are associated with survival time, incidence of multiple primary malignancies, rate of recurrence of primary lesions, and extent of local tumors and metastases.

In animal studies, selenium supplements have been found to protect animals from spontaneous and chemically induced cancers.[14]

None of the researchers responsible for the studies which demonstrate a role for selenium in the prevention of cancer believes selenium is the "cure" or the "answer" to cancer, but they do believe that selenium levels in the diet are definitely a factor. They also recommend that people make dietary changes which would add selenium to their diet, especially if they live in areas where selenium is low in the soil and food supply.

Selenium and Toxic Metals

Selenium has demonstrated the ability to protect animals from the toxic effects of many common pollutants, including mercury, cadmium, silver, thallium, lead, and copper.[15]

REQUIREMENTS FOR SELENIUM

The adult RDA for selenium is 50 micrograms (.05 mg.). The average American diet is believed to contain about 60 micrograms of selenium, but the average diets in areas where heart disease and cancer are low is more like 100 micrograms, about twice the RDA.[16] Several epidemiological studies of selenium bioavailability in soils, selenium blood levels, and levels of glutathione peroxidase have demonstrated that many people may be receiving suboptimal levels of the mineral. Furthermore, evaluations of processed foods have revealed that even some normally high selenium foods become poor sources of the mineral after processing. Boiling, for example, can remove selenium from vegetables.[17]

TOXICITY OF SELENIUM

Like most other trace minerals, selenium can be toxic in excess amounts. Toxic effects, however, would not be expected to occur unless long-term consumption was over 2000 micrograms a day. This is about six to seven times the supplemental amount recommended by some doctors and researchers. In mice, the toxic dose of selenium is 100 to 300 times the required dose.[18]

Naturally occurring selenium toxicity has been reported in

humans and livestock in areas where selenium exists in super-high levels in soil and vegetation.[19]

In the only study to test the effects of selenium supplementation on humans, 500 micrograms of selenium produced no side effects or toxic reactions.[20]

SOURCES OF SELENIUM

The richest natural sources of selenium are organ meats, seafood, whole grains, and brewer's yeast. Special yeasts are available which are grown on a selenium-rich medium. These yeasts actually supply what might be termed supplemental amounts of selenium, and are usually available only in tablet form. Selenium is available in other forms (sodium selenite, for one) in supplements. But tests have shown that selenium which is organically bound to yeast is the most efficiently absorbed source.[21]

29

Silicon

Who would have imagined that *sand* could contain an important factor in maintaining optimum health? Who would guess that the most abundant mineral on earth could be considered a factor in aging, wound healing, and heart disease?

We're talking about silicon. All living tissue contains at least traces of it. It's present in rocks, dust, clay, glass, water, and, of course, sand. And human blood contains the same concentrations of silicon as sea water (1 to 5 ppm).

Yet though silicon shows up in just about every script, no one suspected it was a star performer until quite recently. Because it's present in just about everything, it took really painstaking research methods to provide a silicon-deficient diet. When such a diet was finally devised and maintained, silicon was found to be required for proper growth and development, and supplements of the mineral were found to boost growth and health of test animals significantly.

Silicon's primary function seems to be to help develop and maintain the structural and functional integrity of connective tissue and bone. The "ground" substance or matrix of bone and any collagenous tissue is largely composed of substances called *mucopolysaccharides.* Silicon is known to be an essential component of these substances, and is also thought to help form the connections among the mucopolysaccharides and the structural proteins. So not only is silicon necessary for the "architecture" of the bones and connective tissue, but for the functional strength, too. To get an idea of how important silicon is to health, it's only necessary to run down the list of tissues where silicon is found in high concentrations: bone, blood vessels (especially the aorta), heart, muscle, skin, hair, cartilage, ligaments, liver, lung, and brain.

Silicon (and the mucopolysaccharides) is also essential to healing, the regulation of the transfer of nutrients and water in connective tissue membranes, and embryonic development.[1]

A deficiency of silicon in animals produces depressed growth, pallor, and deformed and brittle bones. No experiments have been performed to reveal the effects of a silicon deficiency in humans. And since silicon has been identified as an essential nutrient so recently, no specific symptoms have been attributed to a lack of the mineral. Nonetheless, there has been some research which suggests that silicon may play a role in healing, heart disease, and aging.

Silicon and Aging

Embryonic and rapidly growing tissues have far higher mucopolysaccharide and silicon concentrations than adult or aging tissues. The aorta, skin, and thymus gland experience particularly marked decline in silicon as they age in many species of animal. In humans, silicon declines with age in the aorta and the skin.[2] Does this mean that increasing the silicon in the diet will retard aging? There is no evidence, in either animals or people, that this is so. But if silicon and the mucopolysaccharides are so vital to the structural and functional integrity of the connective tissue, it's not unreasonable to speculate that keeping silicon levels high might contribute to retarding some of the effects of aging. But "contribute to" is a long way from "completely prevent." So many factors contribute to aging that it's really foolish to believe any single item could make a significant difference if all the other factors are ignored.

Silicon and Healing

For healing to take place, new tissue must be formed over the lesion. This, of course, requires growth of and linking among new elements of tissue "ground substance." Silicon, as a vital component of this ground substance *and* the links, is naturally a factor in healing. Since silicon is so new to the list of essential nutrients, there isn't much research on the effects of supplementation on wound healing. There have been a few reports, however. In one, an extract of cartilage, high in silicon, was used to accelerate wound healing (twenty to forty percent improvement) of surgical patients and dental patients.[3] In another, silicon supplements improved healing in eighty-five percent of a group of people with peptic ulcers who had not responded to conventional therapy.[4]

Silicon and Heart Disease

There appears to be a relationship between silicon and heart disease, although as with all other nutrients, don't assume that this single substance can offer complete protection.

Nevertheless, silicon is found in high concentrations in the arterial wall. These concentrations decline with age, and are even more reduced in atherosclerotic arteries. To make the case even more intriguing, a study of coronary heart disease in Finland found that silicon levels in drinking water were low where heart disease was high, and vice versa. Because certain kinds of food fiber are not only especially high in silicon but also associated with decreased risk of heart disease, some researchers have proposed that the silicon in the fiber is the "active" ingredient.[5]

Doctors have also successfully treated some of the symptoms of heart disease with a high-silicon substance called *chondroitin sulfate*, or CSA. A group of 120 heart patients who had not responded to other forms of treatment were divided into two equal groups. One group received supplements of CSA every day; the others received standard care. Of the supplemented group, four had heart attacks and four died over the course of the six-year study. Out of the other group, however, twenty-four had heart attacks and fourteen died. Patients given CSA also experienced improvement in some symptoms, such as angina, exercise tolerance, and well-being.[6]

REQUIREMENTS AND SOURCES FOR SILICON

No RDA for silicon has been determined. Because silicon is so abundant, a diet of natural foods would most likely supply plenty of this mineral. However, few people subsist on a diet of natural foods. By removing the fibrous portion of grain and refining sugar beets and cane, most of the available silicon is removed. Muscle and organ meats are generally low in silicon, although connective tissue, bones, and skin are high. Beer happens to be a good source of silicon, too.[7] Silicon is available in various supplemental forms, and is sometimes included in multimineral supplements. No toxicity from silicon has been reported.

30

Sodium

Like phosphorus, sodium is a very important, yet very dangerous, mineral. Also, like phosphorus, sodium is dangerous mainly because modern food technology insists on adding sodium compounds to processed and manufactured foods.

Sodium's primary purpose is to help "pump" fluids and nutrients in and out of the cells and cell membranes. The fluid outside the cells contains most of the body's sodium. In normal concentrations, sodium is absolutely essential to the functioning of the cells and, of course, the body. A deficiency can lead to headaches, muscular cramps, weakness, and collapse of the blood vessels. Such a deficiency is quite rare, since most people consume many times the required amount (5 grams is considered a *liberal* allowance).

When dietary sodium is too high, the concentration of the mineral in the fluid surrounding the cells also rises. Small changes in sodium concentrations in the extracellular fluid can markedly raise blood pressure. Some people seem to be more susceptible to this effect than others, but most people appear to be susceptible to some degree. There is evidence that dietary potassium can offer some protection against the blood pressure-raising effect of sodium. (See Potassium chapter.)

To avoid excess sodium in the diet, avoid processed foods. A glance at the labels of processed foods will tell you how really dangerous many of them are. Salt substitutes containing potassium salts will both lower sodium intake and raise potassium intake.

31

Zinc

Perhaps more than any other mineral, zinc demonstrates that a mineral can be as versatile and as important as a vitamin when it comes to creating and maintaining optimum health. Zinc has been identified as a cofactor in at least forty different enzyme systems, covering *every* major physiological function dependent upon enzymes. Without adequate zinc, for example, carbon dioxide exchange in the cells could not take place at a fast enough rate to sustain life.

Zinc also appears to have a major role in the synthesis of nucleic acids, including RNA and DNA, and in protein synthesis. It is necessary for cell growth and the formation of connective tissue, both of which processes depend heavily on nucleic acids and protein synthesis.[1]

Zinc also appears to have a protective role in the cells and cell membranes, perhaps by exerting an antioxidant effect. Metabolism of other minerals, such as copper, magnesium, manganese, and selenium have also been found responsive to changes in zinc balance in the body. In this respect, zinc may perform some regulatory functions.[2]

WHAT HAPPENS WHEN ZINC DEMAND EXCEEDS SUPPLY?

Since zinc is necessary for cell growth, any tissue which depends on relatively rapid cell proliferation will suffer the effects of a deficiency first and most severely. So a zinc deficiency can result in delayed healing of wounds, deformities in offspring born to deficient mothers, impaired development of bones, muscle, and nervous system, delayed sexual maturation, testicular atrophy and dysfunction, loss of hair, deformed nails, skin lesions, infertility, impaired immune response, reduced salivation, atrophy of the thymus gland, and reduced absorption of nutrients.[3]

Zinc deficiency in children will manifest itself in loss of appetite, loss of the sense of taste and smell, impaired growth, dermatitis, diarrhea, hair fall, and depression.[4] *Acrodermatitis enteropathica* is a fatal disease now known to be due to an inherited defect which causes impaired absorption of zinc. The resultant severe deficiency causes diarrhea, loss of hair, severe dermatitis, lesions in the eyes, psychological disturbances, and greatly increased susceptibility to infections. The disease usually appears in early infancy, although breast-fed babies with the disease are protected until they are weaned (breast milk contains zinc which is absorbed extraordinarily efficiently). A child with acrodermatitis enteropathica fails to thrive and is beset with numerous infections. Victims rarely survive childhood. Women surviving into childbearing have given birth to severely deformed infants, owing to their severe zinc deficiency.[5]

Once it was discovered (by accident) that this disease resulted from interference with zinc metabolism, doctors started treating patients with zinc. Several encouraging results were obtained, and now the defect and all its symptoms can be overcome in many persons with administration of as little as 1 to 2 mg. of zinc per kilogram of body weight per day.[6]

A zinc deficiency resulting from inadequate diet can cause symptoms identical with acrodermatitis enteropathica. In several Middle Eastern countries, retarded sexual development and even dwarfism have been found and successfully treated in many people with severe zinc deficiencies.[7]

In adults, zinc deficiency results in the same symptoms as in children, with some differences owing to advanced maturity. For example, whereas young males and females will suffer retarded sexual development, adults will suffer infertility and impaired sexual function. Skin lesions, impaired wound healing, loss of appetite, taste, and smell, hair fall, and increased susceptibility to infection affect all ages in a zinc deficiency.

Zinc and Stress

Like many vitamins, zinc seems to be involved in the body's response to stress. In animal experiments, zinc supplements markedly reduced the number of stress ulcers produced during extreme stress.[8] In human studies, blood levels of zinc have been found to rise considerably in anxious anticipation of stress and during the stress itself (such as surgery). Anesthetic drugs were found to depress zinc levels in the blood, however. Since adrenocortical secretion also rose before and during stress, and was likewise reduced by anesthetics, doctors believe zinc is, like adrenocortical hormone, part of the body's response to stress. Excretion of zinc has also been found to increase by a factor of three to five during stress, another indication that the body prepares to deal with stress by increasing the amount of zinc that's available to tissues for healing or any other purpose zinc has in the body.[9]

Zinc and Infection

In humans, as well as animals, zinc deficiency impairs the body's resistance to infection.[10] Researchers have identified zinc as an antibacterial agent in prostatic fluid, possibly playing a major role in protecting the prostate as well as the rest of the genitourinary system against infection.[11] And topical application of zinc sulphate has been shown to prevent recurrence of genital herpes infection in seven out of ten women.[12]

No studies have been performed with zinc similar to those which have demonstrated an illness-reducing effect of vitamin C. Nonetheless, when zinc deficiencies are corrected, resistance to infections usually improves.

Zinc and Healing

The idea of using zinc to improve healing is not new. The ancient Egyptians applied zinc in the form of calamine to aid healing. Zinc's role in healing may be one reason the body increases zinc blood levels in anticipation of stress. Studies have also found that burns can rapidly drain the body of zinc. Where does the zinc go? Into the burn sites and the fluid surrounding the burn sites, because that is the site of rapid cell growth for reconstruction of burned tissue.

A zinc deficiency can severely impair healing, tests with animals and humans have shown. Several studies have found the incidence of zinc deficiencies to be extremely high in hospital patients with wounds that refuse to heal, or wounds that heal and then reopen. This fact is not so remarkable, since nutrient deficiencies would be expected to interfere with normal bodily functions. What is remarkable is that zinc in excess of "requirements" can *accelerate* healing.

In one study, twenty surgical patients were divided into two groups. One group received zinc supplements three times a day while the other group did not. Though the zinc-supplemented group had larger wounds, their wounds healed in only forty-five days (on the average) while the group that received no zinc took an average of eighty days.[13]

In another study, zinc supplements enabled a group of women undergoing gynecological surgery to go home from the hospital in less than half the time it took women not receiving zinc. The women who received zinc supplements before their surgery (220 mg. zinc sulfate, three times a day) went home eighteen days after their operations. Women not receiving zinc went home thirty-seven days after their operations.[14]

From these results, it appears that zinc supplements might be a good idea for someone planning to undergo surgery, and perhaps for anyone who has a wound that needs healing, even something as minor as a mouth sore. Dentists have reported fifty to a hundred percent reduction in the recurrence of "oral ulcers" after zinc supplementation.[15]

Zinc and Acne

Zinc can also help heal acne. Blood levels of zinc have been found to be significantly lower than normal in men with acne.[16] And when healthy male volunteers were placed on a zinc-deficient diet for three weeks, they developed acne and dry skin. One of the men's acne was quite severe. But zinc supplementation alleviated the symptoms in all men.[17] In one study, zinc supplements twice a day (200 mg. zinc sulfate, equal to 45 mg. zinc) resulted in significant improvement in people with moderate-to-severe acne vulgaris.[18] In another study, supplements of vitamin A and zinc also resulted in improvement; however, zinc alone brought about as much improvement as the combined supplement. The researchers theorized that because zinc is involved in making vitamin A available to the tissues, the healing effect of zinc on acne may be due to the increase in available vitamin A as well as zinc's own effect on healing.

Zinc and Rheumatoid Arthritis

There has been only one report of the use of zinc in rheumatoid arthritis. Basing his therapy on reports that blood levels of zinc are lower than normal in people with rheumatoid arthritis, on the known anti-inflammatory properties of zinc, and on the theory that zinc is in some way involved in the maintenance of the synovial membrane (which becomes inflamed in arthritis) a doctor gave zinc supplements (50 mg. of zinc, three times a day) to arthritis patients for twelve weeks, then gave some a placebo while continuing the zinc therapy in others. The people who received zinc were reported to "fare better" with regard to joint swelling, morning stiffness, walking time, and subjective impressions of overall disease activity.

The doctor who carried out this study was very careful *not* to give the impression that zinc was a *cure* for rheumatoid arthritis. He did acknowledge, however, that his results "suggest that zinc supplementation may offer significant alleviation of many of the symptoms of active rheumatoid arthritis."[19]

Zinc and Heart Disease

Blood plasma levels of zinc have been found to fall within the first three days after a heart attack. The severity of that fall, and the subsequent blood levels of zinc, were found to correlate with the severity of heart disease and the likelihood of survival. As zinc levels were lower, potentially fatal disturbances of the heart rhythm became more severe. And among the patients who survived, higher blood levels of zinc were associated with a shorter hospital stay and a faster recovery.[20]

Zinc supplements were reported to help a small group of people with "severely symptomatic atherosclerotic disease." The blocked blood vessels were interfering with circulation in their arms and legs, making normal activities difficult or impossible. Some of the people had been recommended for surgery or even amputation. After zinc supplementation, their doctors reported substantial improvement which not only allowed them to avoid surgery, but also to go back to their normal everyday activities. One man, for example, had been in line for amputation. But after zinc therapy, he was able to go back to work as a farmer.[21]

Zinc and Sickle Cell Anemia

People with sickle cell anemia have been found to have lower-than-normal blood levels of zinc. They also exhibit some of the symptoms of zinc deficiency, particularly retarded sexual maturation. Early tests with zinc revealed that zinc can significantly diminish the number of blood cells that become "sickled." Zinc can also reduce the number of red blood cells that are already damaged by sickling. The next step was to test the effect of zinc supplements on people with the disease. Zinc supplements (150 mg. of zinc, divided into equal doses given every four hours) were found to improve the anemia in sickle cell patients moderately, *and* to reduce significantly the number and frequency of crippling episodes of pain suffered by sickle cell patients. The average frequency of pain episodes was cut to slightly more than one-third of the previous frequency. Furthermore, retarded sexual maturation was reversed in many of the young men.[22]

Zinc and Male Sexuality

A group of Chicago doctors has made use of zinc supplements to reduce the inflammation of prostatitis. Out of a group of nineteen patients with benign prostatic hypertrophy, supplements of 100 to 150 mg. zinc sulfate, four times a day, resulted in shrinkage of the prostate in fourteen out of the nineteen men. Zinc therapy also increased the concentrations of zinc in the semen, an indication that the increased zinc intake was finding its way to the prostate gland. In a larger group of men with chronic abacterial prostatitis, zinc therapy relieved symptoms in 140 of 200 patients.[23]

Since zinc is necessary for testicular structure and function, which includes testosterone production, it is understandable that a severe enough deficiency can not only retard development of sexual characteristics in adolescents but also inhibit sexual functioning in an already developed man. Doctors working with men undergoing renal dialysis have found that these men apparently have such deficiencies. Treating uremic men suffering impotence as a side effect of their dialysis resulted in *restoration of potency* as well as increasing testosterone levels to normal.[24] So striking were the results, and so safe is zinc therapy, that some doctors have suggested using zinc as the *first line of treatment for impotence—even in apparently healthy men*—as long as no other cause for sexual dysfunction is known.[25]

In other studies, zinc supplementation has been shown to increase testosterone levels and sperm count.[26]

Zinc and Toxic Substances

Zinc has a protective effect against many common poisons. For example, one of the enzymes in which zinc is a cofactor is responsible for the breakdown of *alcohol*. In tests with animals, zinc supplementation was found almost fully to protect animals from lethal doses of alcohol. Zinc apparently helped the body lower alcohol concentrations in the blood faster, before substantial harm could be done.[27]

Zinc also helps protect against lead poisoning. In a group of workers constantly exposed to toxic levels of lead, zinc and vitamin C supplements were found to reduce their blood concentrations of lead by twenty-five percent while they were still exposed to lead.[28]

Zinc and cadmium are frequently found together in nature. In fact, cadmium is a by-product of zinc mining. Because of the chemical affinity between the two, zinc appears to protect against the toxic effects of cadmium. In animals, zinc supplements prevent the retardation of growth by cadmium. Zinc has also been shown to reduce blood and tissue levels of cadmium.[29] In seafood, zinc accompanies cadmium and apparently protects against the toxic reactions to it. In some areas of the world, there seems to be a correlation between high cadmium-to-zinc ratios in the diet and cardiovascular disease. One of the toxic effects of cadmium is elevated blood pressure.[30]

REQUIREMENTS FOR ZINC

The RDA for zinc is 3 mg. for infants up to five months

old, 5 mg. from five months to one year, 10 mg. for children one to ten, 15 mg. for adults, 20 mg. for pregnant women, and 25 mg. for lactating women.

There are many factors which can reduce the body's zinc status and contribute to a deficiency. Most truly severe deficiencies of zinc are thought to be the result of genetic defects or diseases interfering with zinc metabolism. Acrodermatitis enteropatica is an example. Several diseases also cause low blood levels of zinc, perhaps because of increased requirements. These include alcoholism, atherosclerosis, chronic cutaneous ulcers, cirrhosis, Down's syndrome, dwarfism, lung cancer, leukemia, myocardial infarction, pulmonary infection, tuberculosis, diabetes, hepatitis, uremia, burns, bacterial and viral infections, acute inflammatory diseases, malabsorption syndromes, steatorrhea, blood loss, schizophrenia, and thyrotoxicosis.[31]

Perhaps a more serious problem is the possible marginal deficiency in zinc that many doctors feel occurs quite commonly in many otherwise well-nourished populations around the world.[32] Several researchers calculated the amount of zinc provided by a number of average diets and found that many Americans and Canadians may be marginally deficient.[33] Specific groups of people in whom these deficiencies have been found by researchers include infants, preschool and school-age children, teenage and college women, pregnant women, vegetarians, and the elderly.[34] Researchers were surprised to find that eight percent of the middle-class children over four years old in Denver were deficient in zinc severely enough to have diminished or absent senses of taste and smell, poor growth rates, and loss of appetite.[35]

Zinc deficiencies have a way of turning up in the places where zinc is most needed. For example, many infant formulas have been found to have inadequate zinc levels. All infants need zinc for growth and development, of course, but male infants appear to have an increased need, perhaps because of the role zinc plays in male sexual development. In a study of the effects of zinc supplementation of infant formula, male infants responded with increased growth rates while females grew at presupplemental rates.[36]

Hospital patients are the last people who should have inadequate zinc levels, since zinc is necessary for healing. Yet hospital patients happen to be one of the groups of people to be *especially likely* to have zinc deficiencies. In the wound-healing experiments described above, many of the patients were deficient in zinc. Analyses of some hospital meals have found they do not supply the RDA for adults, not to mention extra amounts which are required for speedy healing.[37] Zinc has also been found low in dining-hall meals collected from fifty colleges.[38]

Much of the soil in the United States is apparently deficient in zinc. Deficiencies in zinc have been found in plants in at least thirty states.[39] If the zinc isn't in the food, it can't get into the body through a diet, no matter how "balanced" it is! Modern high-technology farming, which uses synthetic fertilizers and pesticides rather than organic methods, is notorious for not returning adequate quantities of minerals to the soil.

Other factors can affect zinc levels besides disease and deficient food. Zinc absorption varies from twenty to eighty percent, but is normally only twenty to thirty percent. Increased absorption occurs during a deficiency, as the body tries to allow more zinc into the blood. Content of the diet, irrespective of the amount of zinc, can also have an effect. High-fiber diets have been shown to decrease zinc absorption. Apparently, phytates (phosphorus compounds) in cereal grains can inhibit the absorption of zinc. For this reason, zinc from animal foods (which are low in fiber and phytates) contain zinc which is more "available." Just how much fiber in cereals and vegetables affects zinc absorption is not precisely known. Some studies have even shown that there is no effect! In any case, the fact that fiber may decrease zinc absorption is no reason to cut down on fiber, since fiber is every bit as important to our health as zinc, if for different reasons.[40] Lemon juice has also been found to impair zinc absorption.[41] And high protein diets may increase zinc requirements.[42]

Several drugs can cause zinc deficiency, too, including chelating agents, diuretics, corticosteroids, and oral contraceptives.[43]

Cadmium toxicity is prevented by zinc. Cadmium, however, also uses up zinc in the process. So a high-cadmium diet will increase zinc requirements. Unfortunately, food processing and refinement remove zinc, but leave in or increase the cadmium in foods. So a diet of processed foods, in itself, can increase your zinc requirements.[44]

TOXICITY OF ZINC

Zinc is relatively nontoxic with respect to other minerals, because the body has a very efficient mechanism for regulating zinc levels. Absorption is decreased when zinc stores or blood levels are adequate, and elimination of excess zinc occurs rapidly and easily. A single oral dose of zinc in excess of 250 mg. may cause vomiting, which itself is another protective mechanism.[45] Pregnant women, of course, should not overdo *any* supplement.

Excess zinc supplementation may depress blood levels of copper. This effect may be beneficial more often than it is harmful, since many nutritionists and doctors believe copper levels are too high in the diet and drinking water.

The symptoms of zinc toxicity include dehydration, abdominal pain, nausea, lethargy, vomiting, dizziness, and muscular incoordination. Very large quantities of the mineral must be eaten to produce these symptoms, however. Death has been reported after ingestion of 45 grams of zinc sulfate, and after intravenous injection of 7.4 grams of zinc sulfate. A sixteen-year-old boy who ate 16 grams of metallic zinc suffered pronounced lethargy.[46]

In general, zinc is a safe substance. It is even used as an emetic (vomiting inducer) by some doctors. Since the mineral does not accumulate in toxic quantities, most cases of toxicity occur after ingestion of immense quantities. In the studies in which zinc supplements were given, no side effects were reported after long-term administration of zinc.

SOURCES OF ZINC

The best natural sources of zinc are seafoods (especially oysters and herring), liver, meats, milk, eggs, nuts, legumes, and brewer's yeast. For infants, breast milk is the best source of zinc, since the zinc in breast milk is absorbed so well that it has been used to supply zinc in cases of malabsorption and impaired utilization.[47]

Zinc is also available in supplemental form in various compounds (zinc sulfate, zinc gluconate, etc.). Zinc sulfate is the most common form used in medical experiments, despite the fact that it is a stomach irritant. Zinc acetate is also used, and appears to be less troublesome. If zinc sulfate is used, the supplement can be taken with meals to reduce the chances of stomach upset.

32

Other Minerals

The fifteen minerals discussed thus far are by no means the only ones required by the body. We don't yet know *all* the minerals the body needs to maintain life. Sulfur and chlorine, for example, are involved in some physiological functions. But since no researcher has turned up deficiencies of these minerals in either animals or humans, little is written about them.

Some minerals are required in such minute quantities, yet are so relatively abundant, that painstaking care is needed to establish that the element is required. In order to establish essentiality, a deficiency of the element must be experimentally produced. When a mineral is required in milligram amounts, it's difficult enough to isolate laboratory animals from all sources of it. But when the amounts required are capable of floating in on *dust*, the researcher needs not only persistence and dedication, but skill. Such a scientist was the late Dr. Klaus Schwarz. Dr. Schwarz revealed the essentiality of many of the elements in his trace element nutrition laboratory, including selenium, fluorine, and silicon. Dr. Schwarz's technique was so highly developed that he was even able to determine that cadmium, though a poison in the amounts most people are exposed to, is indeed an essential mineral; that without it, animals suffer ill health. Dr. Schwarz added to the list of essential elements *tin*, which is necessary for growth and tooth development; and *vanadium*, which is required for growth and mineralization. Other researchers established the essentiality for nickel.

Dr. Schwarz was even on the trail of lead and titanium, but he was not yet able to reduce the concentration of the minerals low enough to satisfy himself that the test environment was truly deficient.

How far would he have gone? All we can do is ponder what Dr. Schwarz himself said in considering the same question, which was that he wouldn't stop before "coming to the threshold where only one atom of a specific element would be present for one specific gene in the chromosomes of a cell. I could conceive of this as the ultimate limit for a biological trace element function."[1]

section 3
PARTNERS, OUTLAWS, AND QUESTIONS

33

Bioflavonoids

They're not vitamins and they're not minerals, yet they're undeniably able to help many people move closer to optimum health.

They're *bioflavonoids*.

No one believes they're vitamins, though when they were first discovered to have a role in the permeability of capillaries they were named *vitamin P*. Vitamin P was also used to describe the substance in natural sources of vitamin C (citrus fruit) which seemed to boost the effectiveness of the vitamin C in alleviating some of the symptoms of scurvy. Later, this substance was found to be a *group* of substances, all with the ability to affect capillary permeability. The term "vitamin P" was discarded, and *flavonoids* or *bioflavonoids* is used instead. The three bioflavonoids most commonly used are *rutin, quercetin,* and *hesperidin.* In all, however, there are more than 800 flavonoids distributed in plants.

The principal effect of bioflavonoids is to decrease the

permeability and fragility of the blood vessels, and to constrict the capillaries. Bioflavonoids apparently have a binding or thickening effect on the cement substance which holds the capillary wall together. This increases the capillary's efficiency as a biologic filter.

Bioflavonoids are not really vitamins, but they have been called "semi-essential," because of their apparent sparing effect on vitamin C. The original experiments which "discovered" bioflavonoids found that they could prolong the life of animals with scurvy. This is now thought to result from bioflavonoid's protection of vitamin C from oxidation, rather than from any direct vitamin effect. In tests with guinea pigs (which don't manufacture their own vitamin C), bioflavonoids were found to reverse oxidation of already oxidized vitamin C and make it available to the tissues. Animals given oxidized vitamin C plus bioflavonoids had higher tissue levels of the vitamin than animals given fresh, unoxidized vitamin C.[1]

The fact that bioflavonoids are found with vitamin C in natural sources has given rise to the term "vitamin C *complex*." At the levels of vitamin C found in natural foods, the bioflavonoids are a good thing to have in order to enhance bioavailability of the vitamin. And taking vitamin C supplements with bioflavonoids may increase the amount of vitamin C ultimately made available to the tissues. However, many vitamin manufacturers have taken advantage of this by creating supplements containing synthetic vitamin C with *small* amounts of bioflavonoids included. Marketed as "vitamin C complex," or "vitamin C and natural bioflavonoids," they suggest that the entire supplement is natural and charge double or triple what the individual ingredients might cost separately.

Another physiological effect attributed to bioflavonoids is a decrease in the tendency of blood cells to clump together or aggregate. Blood cell aggregation is undesirable, because it interferes with circulation through the microscopic capillaries and increases the chances of dangerous blood clots. Blood cell aggregation has been found to increase considerably during disease, stress, or trauma. When this "clumping" of blood cells blocks circulation through the capillaries, the adverse effects can range from reduced function in an organ to actual damage to the organ through oxygen starvation. Doctors have found that "clumping" of blood cells also occurs in normal, healthy people as well. Blood cell aggregation has also been accused of intensifying the symptoms of many diseases.[2]

Bioflavonoids have also been found to increase the absorption and utilization of vitamin A,[3] and to "spare" (prevent its oxidation, and increase its availability to tissues) *epinephrine*, the adrenal hormone which stimulates the cardiovascular system.

Because of their beneficial effects on the capillaries, bioflavonoids have been used in the treatment of many diseases characterized by increased bleeding from fragile capillaries, such as vascular disease, allergies, diabetes, and menstrual disorders.

Increased capillary fragility is higher in the elderly, and in people with atherosclerosis, high blood pressure, rheumatoid arthritis, diabetes, and infections. A group of Florida doctors tried the effects of bioflavonoids on the disease symptoms in a group of old people under their care. About sixty-four percent of the 189 people tested had increased capillary fragility. Thirty of the people with capillary fragility were given bioflavonoid supplements (600 mg. per day). Capillary fragility was restored to normal in twenty-seven of them. The doctors also reported that bioflavonoids were used on "little strokes," or minor hemorrhages of the cerebral capillaries. Out of thirteen people treated, nine had no recurrence of strokes. Although no dramatic improvement was noted in rheumatoid arthritis patients treated with bioflavonoids, the doctors did report some improvement in symptoms.

Retinitis (inflammation of the retina, with hemorrhaging) was alleviated and prevented from recurring in eighty-five percent of those treated with bioflavonoids. Retinitis is often a complication of high blood pressure or diabetes. Bioflavonoids also halted severe nose bleeds in a group of old people.[4]

Bioflavonoids have been found to halt intermittent bleeding (spotting) in women taking oral contraceptives.[5] Abnormal uterine bleeding (metrorrhagia and menorrhagia) have also been successfully treated with bioflavonoids. And bioflavonoids can prevent the excessive bleeding that often follows the insertion of an IUD. Bioflavonoids strengthen the capillaries of the uterine lining and prevent unnecessary bleeding. All women noted gradual improvement over two to three months, with the most marked alleviation of symptoms by the third menstrual cycle. These same doctors found that bioflavonoids could relieve pain from varicose veins, hemorrhoids, and leg edema in pregnant women.[6]

Bioflavonoids (1200 mg.) and vitamin C (1200 mg.) were found to markedly relieve vasomotor flushing—hot flashes—in ninety-four menopausal women. The bioflavonoids worked better than estrogen supplements.[7]

Bioflavonoids have also been used to treat people with heart disease and cerebrovascular disease. Out of a group of thirty-two people with various cardiovascular problems, including dizziness, history of heart attack, high blood pressure, and heart failure, twenty-six received some benefit from supplements of vitamin C and bioflavonoids (100 to 1000 mg. of each per day).[8]

The rationale for treating cardiovascular disease with bioflavonoids is that if the strength of the blood vessels can be increased and the tendency of the blood to clump can be decreased, the symptoms of the disease should improve. This is a logical approach; however, few researchers followed up on the original experiments carried out in the early 1950s.

Bioflavonoids have a documented antiviral activity. Animals treated with bioflavonoids are better able to resist viral infections.[9] Daily treatment with bioflavonoids (1000 mg.) and vitamin C (1000 mg.) has been found to be effective in speeding the healing of herpes sores on the lips. Presumably, the bioflavonoids increase the resistance of the membranes to penetration by the viruses.[10]

Bioflavonoids have also proved effective in protecting animals against frostbite injury.[11]

SOURCES OF BIOFLAVONOIDS

Bioflavonoids are found in the leaves, stems, flowers, fruits, and roots of most plants. The bioflavonoids which are used in treating diseases—because they are the most active in the body—are the *citrus* bioflavonoids. The white rind of the orange (and other citrus fruits) is especially rich in bioflavonoids. Because bioflavonoids depend on light for their formation, outer parts or leaves of plants generally have the highest concentrations.

Bioflavonoids are available in supplemental form as *rutin* or bioflavonoids, in doses up to 1000 mg.

There is no known toxicity to these substances.

34

The Outlaw Vitamins: B$_{15}$, B$_{17}$, Q, and U

The four substances in this chapter are called the "outlaw vitamins" because none of them has been recognized as a vitamin. One of them, B$_{17}$ (laetrile), has actually been outlawed by the Federal Government.

B$_{15}$

B$_{15}$—also called *pangamic acid* or *pangamate*—has not been shown to be essential to health. No experiments have been performed which demonstrate that a lack of this substance adversely affects health. Because a great variety of beneficial effects have been reported, a lot of people refer to it as a vitamin.

The whole phenomenon of B$_{15}$ (and B$_{17}$) could be referred to as "vitamin hysteria." The substance is being granted more credit than it deserves, and in some cases more credit than *any* substance deserves. This immediately provokes scientists and nutritionists and doctors into coming down on the substance harder than it really deserves. So its defenders become even more enthusiastic. Hence, "vitamin hysteria."

B15 has been credited with beneficial effects in heart disease, muscle fatigue, aging, senility, diabetes, gangrene, high blood pressure, glaucoma, alcoholism, drug addiction, autism, schizophrenia, liver diseases, minimal brain dysfunction, allergies, dermatitis, neuralgia, sciatica, and neuritis. It's supposed to perform all these wonders by extending the lifespan of the cell, improving oxygenation of the blood, stimulating the immune response, facilitating energy metabolism, detoxifying pollutants, synthesizing protein, and regulating blood levels of hormones.[1]

Sounds like a multivitamin-mineral supplement rolled into one substance!

One of the "problems" with B15 is that practically all of the actual research with the substance has been performed and published by Russian nutritionists. Although Russian science was good enough to put the first satellite in orbit and the first man in space, many doctors feel their science isn't reliable when it comes to nutrition and health. Of course, whenever *anyone* publishes or reports something that disagrees with established medical or nutritional attitudes or dogma, the first reaction of most doctors and nutritionists is simply to deny that the work is valid. This allows it to be ignored. And, of course, the fact that the Russians are *the Russians* makes it that much easier to treat everything they say or do with suspicion.

A German doctor published a report of his use of B15 (90 to 180 mg. per day) to treat liver damage, angina pectoris, and psychosomatic syndromes. B15 improved appetite and diuresis in the hepatitis patients, suppressed pain and anxiety in the angina patients, and eliminated many of the psychosomatic problems.[2] There is no mention of any comparison of the effects of B15 and a placebo treatment, however. Often, any new treatment will demonstrate measurable and significant beneficial effects simply because of psychological factors. A "control" group of patients who receive placebo treatments is usually included in a study in order to see just how great the placebo factor is. This is not to say that psychological effects are not valid. There's no doubt that a person's mind can determine many physiological conditions. Yet for the purposes of finding out whether a substance really can have any benefit in treating or preventing illness, you want to account for effects which really aren't due to any properties of the substance itself.

New York physician Allan Cott has reported that B_{15} has proved of benefit in treating children with severe disorders in learning, behavior, and communication (autism).[3]

Natural sources of B_{15} include brewer's yeast, seeds (sunflower, etc.), sprouts, liver, and whole grains. Because it's found in many of the same foods as B vitamins, it's called B_{15}. Its chemical name, pangamic acid, refers to the fact that it's found in seeds *(gamete)*. B_{15} is available in supplemental form in a wide range of doses.

The Food and Drug Administration does not believe B_{15} should be allowed on the market. This may be "vitamin hysteria" on their part. FDA spokespeople have been quoted as saying, "The problem with this kind of quackery is that people who take the pills don't drop dead."[4] That statement suggests that the response of the FDA is more the emotional response of a domineering bureaucratic institution feeling threatened than it is the calm, careful response of an agency that wishes to protect the public from real dangers in the food and drug supply. B_{15} is not a danger, in itself, to anyone's health. It is not a very toxic substance, certainly no more toxic than any vitamin.

The "problem" with B_{15} is in statements like "B_{15} is the secret of good health." A lot of the publicity for B_{15} fosters the attitude that taking the substance can be a "shortcut to good health."

There are no secrets of good health. And there certainly are no shortcuts. Anyone who believes any substance or group of substances can be a shortcut to good health is setting himself up for profound disappointments. (And for a waste of money. B_{15} usually sells for double, triple—or more—the price of any other single nutritional supplement.) Your budget may be able to afford the expense, but your health cannot afford the attitude that taking this or that pill will make up for all the negative influences on health, make up for not doing all the other things you should be doing to maintain health.

B_{17}

B_{17} is more commonly known as *laetrile*. Laetrile *is* an outlaw, since the FDA won't allow its use in the United States. Laetrile's principal component is *amygdalin,* a substance naturally occurring in several plants (vetches, clovers, sorghums, cassava, lima beans, acacia) and in the pits of edible fruits and berries. All the controversy, of course, involves disputed claims over laetrile's anticancer effectiveness and safety. Proponents claim laetrile selectively kills tumor cells while not harming normal cells. Laetrile also contains *cyanide,* which most proponents believe is the active ingredient. The opposition says cyanide is responsible for toxicity, and makes laetrile a dangerous substance. This has been the basis for the FDA's outlawing laetrile. Although various writers will refer to laetrile as a vitamin and say that cancer may be a manifestation of a deficiency of the vitamin, few really believe B_{17} is an essential nutrient, or that it's a nutrient at all, for that matter. Calling it a vitamin was mainly a ploy to get around the FDA's stricter controls on *drugs.*

The true question isn't whether or not laetrile or B_{17} or amygdalin is a vitamin, but whether it is an effective anticancer drug. Unfortunately, a form of vitamin hysteria occurs in this case, too. The Establishment (doctors, drug companies, cancer researchers) does not particularly like the idea that this substance which isn't a result of their work may allegedly have benefit. Their first reaction is to deny, then to ignore. Proponents react by becoming more insistent and vociferous. The cycle continues; the level of accusation, devotion, enthusiasm, and denial intensifies. Hysteria: no one can get a straight answer from anyone.

Proponents of laetrile are probably pushing too hard; the substance probably does have some value as a cancer drug, but is not the "magic bullet" everyone would like to see developed. On the other hand, the opponents may be pushing too hard, too; the climate in cancer research does not encourage—and is actually quite hostile toward—any *new* ideas. Researchers who discover benefit in places where the Cancer Establishment is not looking usually cannot get their work published in medical journals.

Most of the everyday application of these new developments—which are not cures by any means, but perhaps less violent and slightly more effective than conventional methods—goes on quietly, in private offices. Doctors who use frowned-upon therapies for cancer and some other "controversial" diseases have learned to keep their successes quiet if they want to continue practicing in peace.

When the National Cancer Institute caved in and solicited case studies and information from 385,000 doctors, 70,000 health professionals, and pro-laetrile groups, they received only ninety-three cases for evaluation. Out of the ninety-three, only six reports of benefit were judged to be attributable to laetrile.[5] These results suggest that the people who are using laetrile either have nothing significant to report or that they're keeping it a secret.

In 1973, a study of laetrile's effectiveness in treating cancer in animals was performed. A news "leak" that the laetrile-treated animals had less than one-fourth as much cancer as the controls was reported and confirmed in preliminary reports. But the results of the entire study were never published and the investigators decided not to research the problem any further. No *negative* results were ever published. Other investigators have published negative results, however.[6]

Laetrile is toxic. The contention that the cyanide in laetrile attacks only cancer cells is unfounded. Several deaths have been reported in children accidentally eating their parent's laetrile tablets. Other reports of toxicity stem from overindulgence in natural sources of amygdalin, such as apricot kernels and cassava beans.[7]

Of course, if laetrile is an effective cancer drug, its toxicity is a factor only insofar as it is more or less toxic than other anticancer drugs. Most anticancer drugs are *quite* toxic.

Laetrile is legal in a number of states: Alaska, Indiana, Florida, Kansas, Arizona, Nevada, Texas, Washington, Louisiana, New Hampshire, Oklahoma, Delaware, New Jersey, Oregon, and Illinois (at this writing). Legalization may result in a slight relaxation of the hysteria, enough to allow some real clinical evidence (one way or the other) to emerge. One researcher, however, implied that the hysteria would continue because people are dissatisfied with the medical profession's inability to cure cancer and the medical profession is defensive because of that failure. The authors concluded that if laetrile were shown to have anticancer effects, the political, ideological, economic, and medical implications would be "far-reaching and profound."[8]

VITAMIN Q

Vitamin Q is an "outlaw" in the sense that it hasn't been recognized as a vitamin, except by the researcher who discovered and named it, Dr. Armand J. Quick. Dr. Quick maintains that vitamin Q, a substance extracted from soybeans, is involved in the normal clotting of the blood. Dr. Quick has reported beneficial results with the substance in the treatment of the hereditary bleeding disorder *telangiectasia*, in which bleeding is caused by a failure of the blood to clot quickly enough.[9]

No vitamin hysteria is likely in the case of vitamin Q, since Dr. Quick is the first to announce that no one, except the people he treated who had hereditary disorders, needs supplements of vitamin Q.

Actually, further work must be performed before vitamin Q is confirmed as a vitamin. Often a substance will be suspected of being a new vitamin until it's discovered to be an old vitamin showing up in a new source or a new physiological role. The work necessary to sufficiently isolate the substance Dr. Quick calls vitamin Q has not been performed.

VITAMIN U

Vitamin U gets its name from the disease it's supposed to cure: ulcers. In the 1940s, an American physician, Dr. Garnett Cheney, started testing the effects of raw cabbage juice on gastrointestinal ulcers. In animals and in humans, Dr. Cheney's results were consistent: cabbage juice *always* reduced pain and remarkably accelerated healing of ulcers. His final study, which Dr. Cheney did not live to complete, involved testing the effects of raw cabbage juice (extract from the juice of one quart of pressed cabbage) against the effects of a placebo treatment. Once again, cabbage juice resulted in a striking acceleration of healing.[10]

When Dr. Cheney died, the use of cabbage juice in the treatment of ulcers died with him, at least as far as the United States was concerned. Before his death, Dr. Cheney and his colleagues were trying to extract and isolate and identify the active ingredient in cabbage juice. This was called vitamin U. Whether it was a vitamin is doubtful. Nevertheless, a reliable, consistent isolation could not be made and the research was abandoned.

In other countries, however, vitamin U lives. Studies performed in Britain, Hungary, and Russia confirm the ulcer-healing effect of raw cabbage juice. Pain is relieved by the reduction in acidity, and the ulcers heal in about one-third the usual time.[11]

35

The Eight Most Asked Questions about Vitamins and Minerals

If you've read the previous chapters of this book thoroughly, you're aware that many of the questions in this chapter are at least partially answered there. The following answers reflect my own opinion, formed from reading several thousand research reports in medical and scientific journals and writing hundreds of articles about the relationship between nutrition and health. Naturally, my conversations and friendships with many doctors who use nutrition, as well as my own experiences with vitamins and minerals, also influence these answers.

1. IF VITAMINS AND MINERALS ARE SO IMPORTANT TO HEALTH AND SO EFFECTIVE IN TREATING DISEASE, WHY DON'T DOCTORS USE THEM?

Many doctors *do* use nutrition in their practices. Most don't, though. But it's not because vitamins and minerals aren't effective, but rather because doctors are simply not taught very much about nutrition. Doctors are taught to diagnose and treat disease with drugs, surgery, and other invasive therapies. They are not taught to prevent disease or to treat it with natural therapies. Doctors who do use natural therapies have either developed them on their own, learned them from other doctors, or learned them from other healers who don't necessarily have medical training.

The difference between vitamins and drugs is that vitamins are naturally part of the body, whereas drugs are foreign to the body's chemical composition and function. Drugs *interfere* with normal body processes. This interference may produce a desired therapeutic effect, but it's still an interference and likely to cause side effects. Many thousands of people die every year from legal, doctor-prescribed drugs. No one dies from vitamins. Yet many people are helped back to health by vitamins. People are attracted to vitamin therapy because they see and experience firsthand that drugs are not as safe or effective as doctors pretend they are.

The medical profession would have to change considerably before most doctors embraced nutrition as the real factor in health and disease that it is. Nutrition courses in medical schools are growing in number. But you can't really expect to find nutrition treated with the same reverence and seriousness that drug therapy and surgery are, since most doctors' careers and livelihoods depend on them.

2. HOW DO I KNOW WHICH VITAMINS AND MINERALS TO TAKE?

There are several tests designed to measure the status of various nutrients. Hair analysis, for example, gives some idea of mineral balances. Blood, urine, and tissue levels all can give a *limited* view of vitamin-mineral status, limited because there really is no simple way to determine if nutrients are really getting to the areas of the body that need them. Blood levels of a vitamin may be "normal," while a local deficiency exists in one or more tissues.

What further complicates matters is that deficiencies in only a single nutrient are rare, and there is no reliable uniformity in symptoms of multiple deficiencies. The dietary habits and conditions that lead to deficiencies usually lead to more than one deficiency at a time. And the interdependence of the vitamins and minerals can result in multiple deficiencies stemming from a single deficiency. A deficiency of a B vitamin, for example, can lead to malabsorption of most other nutrients.

Some doctors and nutritionists say that the most prominent symptoms will reveal which nutrient is most acutely deficient. But even in cases where the offending deficiency *is* known, doctors usually give supportive supplements of multivitamins and minerals in addition to extra amounts of the primary nutrient.

Since the deficiency symptoms for every vitamin and mineral are described here, you might well read over this information for hints of any deficiencies you might have. Keep in mind, however, that many of these symptoms have been discovered in people with *severe* deficiencies. A marginal deficiency will cause less acute symptoms.

3. HOW MANY VITAMINS AND MINERALS SHOULD I TAKE?

When nutritionally oriented doctors were asked this question, the most common answer was to begin with low-dose supplements and increase dosages slowly until you note some beneficial effect. Of course, you may not notice any effect for many weeks. A few doctors asked said they start with high doses and work their way *down*. This is usually the procedure when someone is obviously suffering from severe deficiencies. If you have symptoms of a deficiency, if you *know* your diet is inadequate, or if you're ill, you may want to start at relatively high doses. But if you are healthy, under little stress, and proud of your diet, but want a little "nutritional insurance," you should start with low-dose supplements.

4. HOW DO I BUY SUPPLEMENTS?

Buy supplements the same way you buy anything else: carefully compare and evaluate different brands. There are three ways to buy supplements: through the mail; in health food stores; and in supermarkets, drug stores, and department stores. Raw materials for supplements are supplied by a handful of pharmaceutical companies, so differences in price are attributable only to differences in potency and packaging. So you should not *assume* that the most expensive supplement is any better than the cheapest.

In comparing brands, you should examine exactly what you're getting for your money. Don't assume that a multi-vitamin and mineral supplement necessarily supplies more for your money than individual supplements. A multi-supplement offers a certain amount of convenience, but may contain lower-than-needed amounts of many nutrients. Multi-supplements will usually supply the RDA or slightly better amounts of most nutrients. You may wish to buy individual supplements of the few vitamins or minerals you want to take in larger amounts, such as vitamins C, pyridoxine, E, or calcium, zinc, or iron. In buying B complex supplements, check to see if all eleven vitamins are present. If you want extra large amounts of some of the B complex, it may pay to use individual supplements for those and use a multi-supplement for the rest.

5. ARE NATURAL VITAMINS BETTER THAN SYNTHETIC?

Natural vitamins are supposedly derived from natural sources, i.e., extracted from food. Synthetic vitamins are produced by mimicking natural chemical processes that produce the vitamins. In my years of researching and writing about nutrition, I have come across a lot of suggestions and claims that natural vitamins are superior, but no actual research evidence that can be applied across the board. For example, natural vitamins are said to be better absorbed and utilized. While this may be true for vitamin D, there is no evidence that it is true for any other vitamins.

Some writers have created a lot of copy out of the fact that natural vitamin E bends a beam of light in a different direction from synthetic vitamin E. This is true and fascinating, but I have never heard or read anyone describe *what difference* it makes to the body!

Although natural foods are better than synthetic foods, natural vitamins are not necessarily better than synthetic, because vitamins are distinct compounds. Food is a mixture of *many* diverse compounds, many of which we know little or nothing about. We can't expect to duplicate food and come up with anything remotely resembling the real thing. Processing food removes many of the factors we know are necessary *and* many we know nothing about. A similar argument is used to explain the superiority of natural vitamins—that they contain substances which are necessary for the utilization and absorption of the vitamin, as well as additional undiscovered vitamins. This is an attractive argument, because it is true in certain cases. In nature, vitamin C is usually accompanied by the bioflavonoids. And there probably *are* undiscovered vitamins lurking in natural foods. But that doesn't necessarily mean they're lurking in natural vitamins. The best—and cheapest— way to make sure you're getting all these unknown *and* known substances is to have a good natural diet.

Furthermore, many vitamin supplements labeled "natural" are really synthetic vitamins mixed with some natural sources of the vitamin. Any high potency supplement of B complex or C is made this way, simply because natural sources of these vitamins cannot practically supply doses high enough to be labeled "megadoses." As for the fat soluble vitamins, A, D, and E, natural sources are available which can provide high doses at a price more or less competitive with synthetic vitamins.

One of the myths about natural vitamins is that they're somehow plucked from nature by elves working in a forest somewhere. They're not. They're subject to many of the same manufacturing rituals and errors as any processed food.

6. WHEN SHOULD I TAKE MY SUPPLEMENTS?

The best and most convenient time to take supplements is with meals. The only reason you might not want to take certain supplements with meals is if elements in the food interfered with absorption of the vitamins or minerals, such as might occur in high-fiber diets. However, the only nutrient with which there's evidence of this consistently occurring is zinc. So you might wish to take a zinc supplement with low-fiber meals or before bed. If the zinc supplement is zinc sulfate, however, it's still best taken with meals. Taken alone, zinc sulfate can irritate the stomach.

Some doctors and nutritionists recommend spreading supplements over the day, to maximize absorption and spread out the time when blood levels are high. This makes good sense but may be inconvenient. If you can get into the habit of taking supplements at each meal, fine. If not, take them with one meal or before bed.

7. IF I TAKE VITAMIN AND MINERAL SUPPLEMENTS, DO I STILL HAVE TO WATCH MY DIET?

Of course. There are many things we don't know about nutrition. A purified diet of all known nutrients does not always produce healthy offspring, in animal experiments. So there are obviously a few things we need that only a good diet can provide. Supplements should not be taken to bolster a junk-food diet's shortcomings. No amount of supplementation can make up for the adverse effects of a diet high in fat, sugar, and salt, and low in fresh foods and whole foods. It's better to be conscious and careful of your diet and not take supplements than to rely on supplements and neglect your diet.

8. WILL VITAMIN AND MINERAL SUPPLEMENTS CHANGE MY LIFE?

That depends. If you're now suffering from a deficiency, supplements could very well change your life within days, weeks, or months. There are many things vitamin and mineral supplements can't do, though, so don't expect miracles. There are many more things you can do for yourself. Although it is a big thing, changing your diet for the better is just one of many things. I have yet to hear from someone who has changed his or her diet along the lines implied in this book and not felt better in many ways.

For many people, interest in vitamins and minerals is a first step toward increased consciousness of many aspects of health. Changes in your diet may lead to changes in many of your daily habits. You may find yourself reading more about health and fitness and doing many things you never thought you'd ever do: running, hiking, skiing, walking instead of driving, cycling, yoga postures, growing sprouts, etc. These changes will come about more from *inside you* than from any biochemical reactions wrought by the supplements. You will realize that you *can* have power over your own health, and that your diet is just one area where you can start winning the struggle for optimum health.

Notes

The standard reference works used for much of the basic information about vitamins and minerals were:

1. Burton, B. T. *Human Nutrition,* NY: McGraw-Hill, 1976. (Formerly called *The Heinz Handbook of Nutrition.*
2. *Vitamin Manual,* Kalamazoo, Michigan: The Upjohn Co.
3. Williams, R. J., *Physicians' Handbook of Nutritional Science,* Springfield, Illinois: Charles C. Thomas, 1977.
4. Williams, R. J., *Nutrition Against Disease,* Bantam, 1978.
5. Schroeder, H. A. *The Trace Elements and Man,* Devin-Adair, 1973.
6. Williams, R. J., and Kaleta, D. K. *A Physicians's Handbook of Orthomolecular Medicine,* NY: Pergamon Press, 1978.

I heartily recommend these books for anyone who wishes to extend their knowledge of the fundamental principles of nutrition and vitamin-mineral therapy.

CHAPTER 1   VITAMIN A

1. The American Journal of Clinical Nutrition, Vol. 23, N. 3, pp. 311-29
2. Nutrition Reviews, Vol. 37, N. 2, Feb. 1979, p. 38
3. F.A.S.E.B. Proceedings, 21, 1962, p. 362
   Archives of Otolaryngology, 75, 1962, p. 36
4. The Sightsaving Review, Vol. 48, fall, 1978
5. Opt. J. Rev. Optom., Vol. 100, N. 6, Mar. 15, 1972
6. The Vitamins, Vol. 1, Academic Press, NY, 1967
7. Skin and Allergy News, Sept. 1973
8. Journal of Infectious Diseases, May 1974
9. Journal of Nutrition, Vol., 57, N. 2, 1955
10. Annals of Surgery, Jun. 1975
11. Annals of Surgery, Oct. 1969
12. South African Medical Journal, Feb. 12, 1967
13. Oncology, 33, pp. 183-87, 1977
14. International Journal of Cancer, Vol. 15, 1975
15. Clinical Oncology, 3, pp. 203-7, 1977
16. British Medical J., Dec. 11, 1976, and Jul. 31, 1976
17. Oncology, 33, pp. 183-87, 1977
18. Proc. Amer. Assn. of Cancer Res. (AACR Abstr.), Vol. 18, Mar. 1977
19. Trans. Ophth. Soc. U.K., 1978, 98, p. 128
20. Nutrition Against Disease, Williams, R. J.; pp. 59, 70
21. Physicians' Handbook of Nutr. Science, p. 94
22. J. of Amer. Dietetic Assn., Vol. 70, N. 4, Apr. 1977
23. J. of Nat. Science and Vitaminology, Oct. 1974
24. J. of Amer. Dietetic Assn., Vol. 72, N. 5
25. Vitamin Manual, Upjohn Co.
26. J. of the Internat. Academy of Prev. Medicine, Vol. 5, N. 1, 1978
27. BMJ, Feb. 4, 1978
28. Amer. J. of Surgery, Vol. 95, Mar. 1958
29. Internat. Journal of Vit. Nutr. Res., 47, 1977
30. Internat. Journal of Vit. Nutr. Res., 46, 1976

CHAPTER 2   THIAMINE

1. Biochemical Pharmacology, Vol. 27, pp. 1677-83
2. Neurology, Jul. 1978, p. 691
   Journal of Nutr. Vol. 107, N. 10., Oct. 1977, pp. 1902-8
3. Nutrition Against Disease, p. 109
4. Proc. Soc. Exp. Biol. and Med., 157, 1978, pp. 421-23
5. J. of Applied Nutr. Vol. 29, N. 1&2, Spring, 1977
6. Medical World News, Aug. 8, 1969
7. The Medical Jour. of Australia, Jan. 15, 1977

8. Bulletin of Exp. Biol. and Med.
9. CMA Journal, Vol. 108, Jun. 2, 1973
10. Jour. of Speech and Hearing Disorders, Vol. 14, N. 4, 1951, p. 327
11. F.A.S.E.B. Proceedings, Vol. 37, N. 3, p. 671
12. Pediatric Research, Vol. 11, N. 4, 1977
13. Nutrition Reports Internat., Vol. 12, N. 3, Sept. 1975
14. Jour. of Nutr. Science and Vitaminology, Vol. 22, 1976
15. Jour. of Human Nutr., 30, 1976, p. 333
16. The Amer. Jour. of Clin. Nutr., 30, Oct. 1977
17. Federation Proceedings, Vol. 35, N. 3, Mar. 1976, p. 443
18. Nutr. Reports Internat., May 1974
19. Internat. J. for Vit. Nutr. Res. Vol. 46, 1976
20. Contraception, Vol. 14, N. 3, Sept. 1976, p. 309
21. Jour. of Nutr. 107, 1977, p. 775
22. Medical World News, Oct. 13, 1961
23. Nutr. Metab., 20, 1976, p. 1
24. Internat. J. for Vit. Nutr. Res., 13(2), 1978
25. Jour. of Applied Nutr., Vol. 29, N. 1&2, spring 1977
26. Jour. of Amer. Dietetic Assn. Vol. 57, 1970, p. 436
27. Vitamin Manual, Upjohn, p. 32

CHAPTER 3   RIBOFLAVIN

1. Prog. Fed. Nutr. Science, Vol. 2, 1977, p. 357
2. Nutrition Reviews, Vol. 35, N. 9, Sept. 1977
3. Prog. Fed. Nutr. Science, Vol. 2, 1977, p. 357
4. Nutr. Reviews, Vol. 31, N. 3, Mar. 1973
5. Prog. Fed. Nutr. Science, Vol. 2, 1977, p. 357
6. Nutr. Reports Internat. Vol. 14, N. 3, 1976
7. Internat. Jour. of Vit. Nutr. Res., 46, 1976, p. 422
8. The Lancet, Jan. 7, 1978
9. The Amer. J. of Clinical Nutr., 26, Feb. 1973, p. 150
10. Plant Foods For Man, 2, 1976, p. 53
11. Nutr. Metab., 20:3, 1976, p. 168
12. Nutr. Metab., 20:3, 1976, p. 1
13. Proc. Soc. Exp. Biol. and Med., 157, 1978, p. 421
14. Prog. Fed. Nutr. Science, Vol. 2, 1977, p. 357
15. Modern Medicine, Vol. 47, No. 1, Jan. 15-Jan. 30, 1979
16. Prog. Fed. Nutr. Science, Vol. 2, 1977, p. 357
17. Cancer, Vol. 39, N. 4, 1977
18. Prog. Fed. Nutr. Science, Vol. 2, 1977, p. 357
19. Family Practice News, Vol. 6, N. 1, 1975, p. 5
20. Pediatric Res., Vol. 10, N. 4, Apr. 1976

21. American Heart Journal, Vol. 92, No. 2, Aug. 1976, p. 135
22. Pediatric News, Jul. 1976, Vol. 10, N. 7
23. The Amer. J. of Clin. Nutr., 31, Feb. 1978, p. 247
24. Contraception, Vol. 14, Sept. 1976, N. 3
25. Family Practice News, Vol. 6, N. 1, 1975, p. 5
26. Prog. Fed. Nutr. Science, Vol. 2, p. 357
27. Vitamin Manual, Upjohn
28. F.A.S.E.B. Proceedings, Vol. 37, N. 3, Mar. 1978, p. 756

CHAPTER 4   NIACIN

1. Bibliotheca Nutrio et Dieta, Vol. 24, 1976, p. 32
2. Experientia, 30:8, Aug. 15, 1974
3. Orthomolecular Psychiatry, Vol. 3, N. 4, 1974, p. 280
4. Williams, R. J., and Kaleta, D. K., A Physician's Handbook of Ortho-molecular Medicine: Pergamon Press, NY, 1978
5. Experientia, 30:8, Aug. 15, 1974, p. 32
6. Family Practice News, Vol. 5, N. 17, Sept. 1975
7. CMA Journal, Vol. 108, Jan. 20, 1973
8. Archives of General Psychiatry, Vol. 31, Oct. 1974
9. Medical Tribune, Vol. 19, N. 22, Jun. 21, 1978, p. 19
10. Modern Medicine, Apr. 1, 1974, p. 79
11. Amer. Journal of Surgery, Vol. 93, Mar. 1958, P. 438
12. Journal of the Amer. Med. Assn., Vol. 235, N. 21, May 24, 1976
13. Journal of the Amer. Geriatrics Soc., Vol. III, N. 2, Nov. 1955
14. Nutrition Reviews, Vol. 33, N. 10, Oct. 1975
15. Clinical Res., Vol. 25, N. 3, Apr. 1977
16. Nutrition Reviews, Vol. 33, Oct. 1975
17. Orthomolecular Psychiatry, Vol. 4, N. 4, 1975, p. 297
18. Internat. J. of Vit. Nutr. Res., N. 46, 1976, p. 58

CHAPTER 5   PYRIDOXINE

1. Neurology, Jan. 1978, p. 47
2. Amer. J. of Clin. Nutr. 26, Apr. 1973, p. 420
3. J. Nutr. Science and Vitaminol., 22, 1976, p. 105
4. Vitamins and Hormones, Vol. 22, 1964, p. 677
5. Nutr. Reviews, Vol. 34, N. 6, Jun. 1976
6. Vitamins and Hormones, Vol. 22, 1964, p. 677
7. Amer. Jour. Obstet. Gyn., Vol. 125, N. 8, P. 1063
8. Amer. Jour. Psychiatry, 130:11, Nov. 1973
9. Amer. Jour. Clin. Nutr. Jul. 1973
10. The Lancet, Apr. 10, 1976, p. 7963

11. Contraception, Vol. 6, N. 4, p. 265
12. British Med. Jour., Jul. 5, 1975
13. Amer. J. of Obstet. Gyn., Vol. 127, No. 6, 1977
14. Parade, Aug. 22, 1976
15. Pathology, 9, Apr. 1977, p. 95
16. Aust. & New Zealand Jour. Med., Dec. 1977
17. Jour. Amer. Pod. Assn.
18. Annals Rheum., Dis., 35, 1976, p. 177
19. Amer. Jour. Clin. Nutr. 28, Nov. 1975, p. 1200
20. Physician's Handbook of Orthomolecular Medicine
21. Res. Comm. in Chem. Path. & Pharmacol. Vol. 13, N. 4, Apr. 1976
22. Ellis, John, Vitamin B6, The Doctor's Report, Harper & Row, 1973
23. Ob. Gyn. News, May 1, 1974
24. Ob. Gyn. News, Mar. 15, 1979, p. 2
25. Physician's Handbook of Orthomolecular Medicine
26. Pediatrics, Vol. 55, N. 3, Mar. 1975, p. 437
27. Amer. Jour. Dis. Child., Vol. 132, Aug. 1978
28. Amer. Jour. Psychiatry, 135 (4), Apr. 1978
29. Developmental Med. & Child Neur., Vol. 15, 1973, p. 541
30. The Lancet, Mar. 19, 1977
31. Amer. Jour. Clinical Nutr., 30, Oct. 1977, p. 1677
32. Urology, Dec. 1977
33. Gastroenterology, Vol. 71, No. 5
34. Jour. of Human Nutr., 30, 1976, p. 333
35. Minnesota Medicine, Feb. 1974, p. 81
36. New England Jour. of Med., Vol. 294, N. 17, Apr. 22, 1976
37. Internat. Jour. Vit. Nutr. Res., 48:4
38. Nutr. Reviews, Vol. 34, No. 1, Jan. 1976
39. Shultz, T. D., and Leklem, J. E., Oregon State U., Corvallis
40. Amer. Jour. Clin. Nutr., 29, Aug. 1976, p. 847
41. F.A.S.E.B. Proceedings, Apr. 1974
42. Jour. of Nutr., Vol. 106, N. 7, Jul. 1976
43. Same as footnote N. 39
44. South African Med. Jour., Vol. 49, 12-6-75
45. The Lancet, Nov. 1, 1975, p. 868

CHAPTER 6   FOLATE

1. The Lancet, Oct. 16, 1976, p. 836
2. BMJ, 1, 1976, p. 1176
3. Nutr. Rep. Internat., Vol. 12, N. 3, Sept. 1975
4. Amer. Jour. Clin. Nutr., Vol. 28, Mar. 1975, p. 225
5. Arch. Neurol., Vol. 35, Sept. 1978

6. Jour. of Clinical Psychiatry, 39 (4), April 1978
7. BMJ, 2, 1973, p. 398
8. Southern Med. Jour., Vol. 70, N. 8, p. 919
9. Eur. Neurol., 16, 1977, p. 230
10. CMA Journal, Vol. 115, August 7, 1976
11. The Lancet, August 9, 1975
12. Pediatric Clinics of North America, Vol. 23, N. 3, Aug. 1976, p. 561
13. BMJ, May 15, 1976
14. Southern Med. Jour., Vol. 70, N. 8, p. 919
15. Pediatric Res., Vol. 11, N. 4, p. 518
16. Biochemical Medicine, Vol. 19, p. 260
17. Clinical Res., Vol. 24, N. 3, April 1976
18. Cutis, July, 1977, p. 39
19. Brit. Jour. Dermatol., Vol. 89, 1973, p. 335
20. Skin and Allergy News, Vol. 7, N. 11, Nov. 1976, p. 21
21. Jour. Periodontology, Vol. 47, N. 1, p. 667
22. Jour. Dental Res., Vol. 56, N. 34, 1977
23. IADR Abstracts, N. 958, 1978
24. New England Jour. Med., Sept. 22, 1977, p. 670
25. The Lancet, Feb. 26, 1977, p. 462
26. Archives of Dis. in Childhood, 1977, Vol. 52
27. Jour. of Pediatrics, Dec. 1978
28. Amer. Jour. Obstet. Gyn., Sept. 15, 1977, p. 222
29. Amer. Jour. Obstet. Gyn., Sept. 15, 1975
30. Amer. Jour. Clin. Nutr., June 1, 1971
31. The Med. Jour. of Australia, Sept. 21, 1974, P. 429
32. Amer. Jour. Obstet Gyn., Vol. 128, N. 3, June 1, 1977
33. CMA Jour., Vol. 115, August 7, 1976
34. Internat. Jour. Vit. Nutr. Res., 49, 1979
35. Jour. of Nutr., Vol. 106, N. 7, Jul. 1976
36. Acta Paediatr. Scand., 68, 1979, p. 239
37. Internat. Jour. Vit. Nutr. Res., 46, N. 4., 1976
38. Amer. Jour. Clin. Nutr., Vol. 30, N. 4, Apr. 1977
39. The Lancet, October 4, 1975, p. 640, and Apr. 9, 1977, p. 814
40. Jour. of Human Nutr., 30, 1976, p. 333
    Southern Med. Jour., Aug. 1977
    Brit. Jour. Clin. Pharmacol., 5, 1978, p. 167
41. BMJ, Oct. 18, 1975
42. The Lancet, Dec. 14, 1974, p. 1416
43. Internal Med. News, Vol. 8, N. 7
44. Federation Proceedings, Vol. 37, N. 3, Mar. 1, 1978, p. 493
45. Vitamin Manual, Upjohn Co., p. 47
46. Nutr. Rep. Internat., Apr. 1978
    Jour. Clin Psychiatry, 39(4), Apr. 1978
47. BMJ, Sept. 18, 1976

CHAPTER 7 COBALAMIN

1. Annals of Internal Med., 80, 1974, p. 326
2. Annals of Internal Med., 78, 1973, p. 533
3. Postgrad. Med., 54, 1973, p. 113
4. Amer. Jour. Ophthalmology, Apr. 1977
   BMJ, May 10, 1975, p. 336
   Canadian Jour. Ophthm., 13, 1978, p. 105
5. Internat. Jour. Vit. Nutr. Res., 47, 1977
6. The Lancet, Oct. 16, 1976
7. Acta Medica Scanda., 177, 1965, p. 689
8. CMA Journal, Jan. 24, 1976
9. Clinical Psychiatry News, Mar. 1976
10. Jour. Clinical Psychiatry, Vol. 36, N. 6, 1975
11. Brit. Jour. Nutr., N. 358
12. Blood, Vol. 47, N. 5, 1976
13. Jour. of Applied Nutr.
14. Ob. Gyn. News, Sept. 1, 1977, p. 12
15. Medical News, Jun. 24, 1974
16. Science News, Apr. 7, 1973
17. JAMA, Vol. 231, N. 3, Jan. 20, 1975, p. 289
18. New England Jour. Med., Vol. 299, N. 23, p. 1319
19. Nutr. Reviews
20. Internat. Jour. Vit. Nutr. Res., Vol. 46, N. 4
21. Journal of Human Nutr., 30, 1976, p. 333
22. American Pharmaceutical Assoc., Sept. 1977, p. 585
23. Acta Medica Scand., 200, 1976, p. 309
24. Clinical Research, Vol. 24, N. 3, 1976

CHAPTER 8 BIOTIN

1. The Vitamins, Vol. II, Sebrell & Harris, eds., Academic Press, 1968
2. The Amer. Jour. Clinical Nutr., 30, Sept. 1977 p. 1408
3. Internat. Jour. Vit. Nutr. Res., 47, 1977, p. 107
4. Pediatrics, Vol. 44, 1969
5. Pediatric Clinics of North Amer., Vol. 23, No. 3, Aug. 1976
6. Same as Footnote N. 5
7. Same as N. 3
8. Biotin, Roche Chemical Division, Nutley, N. J. (pamphlet)
9. Same as N. 3
10. Jour. Clinical Pathology, 29, 1976, p. 58

CHAPTER 9 PANTOTHENATE

1. Vitamins and Hormones, Vol. 11, 1953, p. 133
2. J. of Nutr., Vol. 105, N. 1, Jan. 1975

3. Proceedings of the Soc. Exp. Biol. Med., Vol. 86, 1954, p. 693
4. Same as N. 1
5. The Lancet, Oct. 23, 1963, p. 862
6. The Amer. Jour. Clin. Nutr., 29, Dec. 1976, p. 1333
7. Amer. Jour. Surgery, Jan. 1959
8. Acta Paediatrica Hungaricae, Vol. 4, N. 1, 1963
9. Nutrition Against Disease, Williams, R. J.
10. Same as N. 1
11. Same as N. 9

CHAPTER 10   CHOLINE

1. New England Jour. Med., Vol. 300, N. 19, May 10, 1979, p. 1113
2. New England Jour. Med., Vol. 297, N. 10, Sept. 8, 1977, p. 524
3. The Lancet, Oct. 4, 1978, p. 837
4. The Lancet, Oct. 1, 1977, p. 711
5. Life Sciences, Vol. 22, 1978, p. 1555
6. Medical Tribune, Wed., Feb. 8, 1978, P. 17
7. Neurology, Sept. 1977, p. 887
8. Current Therapeutic Res., Vol. 18, N. 3, Sept. 1975
9. Amer. Jour. Clinical Nutr., 2, 1954, p. 396
10. Nutrition Against Disease, Williams, R. J.
11. Jour. National Cancer Inst., 61(3), 1978, p. 813

CHAPTER 11   INOSITOL

1. Jour. Amer. Diabetes Assoc., Vol. 26, Supplement, 1, p. 372
2. Jour. Urology, 59, 1948, p. 595
3. Same as N. 2

CHAPTER 12   PABA

1. Jour. Invest. Dermatology, 65, 1975, p. 543
2. A.M.P. BioResearch Inst. Bulletin, fall 1975

CHAPTER 13   VITAMIN C

1. Amer. Jour. Clin. Nutr., Feb. 1977
2. Nutr. Reviews, Vol. 34, N. 9, Sept. 1976, p. 278
3. Amer. Jour. Clin. Nutr., Vol. 23, N. 3, Mar. 1970, p. 311
4. Nutrition Today, Jan./Feb. 1977, p. 10
5. Comp. Physiol. Ecol., Vol. 3, N. 2, 1978, p. 81
6. Internat. Jour. Fertility, Vol. 22, N. 3, 1977

7. Archives of Disease in Childhood, 51, 1976, p. 944
8. Jour. Applied Physiol., Aug. 1976
9. Nutr. Reports Internat., Vol. 17, N. 3, Mar. 1978, p. 315
10. Arch. Dermatol., Vol. 113, Jan. 1977, p. 91
11. BMJ, Feb. 17, 1979, p. 437
12. Levinson, R. A., and Peterson, C. A., Ophthalmology Dept., Univ. Alabama
13. Same as N. 11
14. Jour. Amer. Diabetes Assn., Oct. 1975
15. Oral Surgery, Vol. 45, N. 1, Jan. 1978
16. The Lancet, Jun. 22, 1968
17. Physician's Handbook of Orthomolecular Medicine, p. 46
18. British Heart Journal, 40, 1978, p. 64
19. Canadian M.A. Jour. (CMA J.), Jul. 1953, Vol. 69, p. 17
20. CMA Jour., 72, Apr. 1955, p. 500
21. Terapeuticheskii Archiv. Vol. 28, 1956, p. 59
22. Internat. Jour. Vit. Nutr. Res., 47, 1977, p. 123
23. Atherosclerosis, 24, 1976, p. 1
24. Nutr. Reports Internat., Vol. 17, N. 2, Feb. 1978
25. The Lancet, May 13, 1975, p. 1055
26. The Lancet, Sept. 17, 1977, p. 611
27. Amer. Jour. Clin. Nutr., Vol. 31, N. 4, Apr. 1978, p. 712
    Diabetes, 27(52), 1978, Abstr. N. 65
28. Atherosclerosis, 30, 1978, p. 351
29. The Lancet, Jan. 31, 1976, p. 247
30. Internat. Jour. Vit. Nutr. Res., Vol. 46, N. 3, 1976, p. 275
31. Diabetes, 27(52), 1978
    Clinical Research, Vol. 26, N. 1, 1978
32. Internat. Jour. Vit. Nutr. Res., 48, 1978, N. 4
33. The Lancet, Jan. 31, 1976
34. Perspectives in Biology and Med., winter, 1974
35. Acta. vitamin. enzymol., 31, 1977, p. 43
    Nutrition Today, Jan./Feb. 1977
36. British Heart Journal, 40, 1978, p. 64
    Internat. Jour. Vit. Nutr. Res., 47, 1977
37. Jour. Allergy Clin. Immunol., Mar. 1978, p. 132
    Experientia, 33(3), 1977
38. Jour. of Surgical Res., Vol. 22, N. 2, Feb. 1977
39. Infect. Immun., 10, 409, 1974
    Experientia, 33(3), 15, 3, 1977
    Acta Pathologica et Microbiol. Scandinavica, Vol. 84, N. 5, 1976
40. Chem-Biol. Interactions, 9, 1974, p. 273
41. Internat. Jour. Vit. Nutr. Res. 47, 1977, p. 248

42. Internat. Jour. Vit. Nutr. Res. 48, 1978, N. 2, p. 159
43. Med. Jour. Australia, Feb. 9, 1974
44. Same as N. 40
45. Cancer Res. 39(3), Mar. 1979, p. 663
46. Oncology, 33, 1976, p. 183
47. Same as N. 45
48. Same as N. 45
49. Same as N. 45
50. Jour. of the Internat. Aca. Preventive Med., Vol. 5, N. 1
51. Chem-Biol. Interactions, 9, 1974, p. 285
52. Chem.-Biol. Interactions, 11, 1975, p. 387
    Jour. of the IAPM, Vol. 5, N. 1
53. Proceedings of the Nat. Acad. Science USA, Vol. 75, N. 9, 1978, p. 4538
    Proc. Nat. Acad. Sci. USA, Vol. 73, N. 10, Oct. 1976, p. 3685
    Jour. IAPM, Vol. 5, N. 1
54. Jour. IAPM, Vol. 5, N. 1, 1978
55. Same as N. 54
56. Jour. IAPM, Vol. 3, N. 1, 1979
57. Medical Tribune, Vol. 18, N. 32, p. 1
58. Cancer Research, 39, 1979, p. 663
59. Same as N. 54
60. Acta. Vitamin. Enzymol., 32, 45, 1978
61. Proceedings of the Nutr. Soc., Vol. 35, N. 3, p. 121A
62. Dry Res., 27(I), N. 6, 1977
63. Experientia, 35/2, 1979, p. 244
64. Physician's Handbook of Ortho. Medicine, p. 78
65. Nutr. Rep. Internat., Vol. 16, N. 1, July 1973
66. Plant Foods For Man, 2, 1976, p. 53
67. Rev. of Czechoslovak Medicine, Vol. 22, N. 4, 1976, p. 209
68. Pediatric News, Vol. 11, N. 11, Nov. 1977, p. 1
69. Jour. Amer. Geriatric Society, Vol. 24, N. 3, 1976
70. Proc. Soc. Exp. Biol. & Med., 154, 1977, p. 146
71. Archives of Environ. Health, Vol. 28, Feb. 1974, p. 105
72. The Amer. Jour. Clin. Nutr., 31, 1978, p. 1491
73. Federation Proceedings, Vol. 37, N. 3, Mar. 1, 1978, p. 405
74. Arch. Environ. Health, Vol. 28, Feb. 1974
75. Internat. Jour. Vit. Nutr. Res., 47, 1977
76. Nutr. Rep. Internat., Vol. 15, N. 2, Feb. 1977
77. The Jour. of Nutr., Vol. 108, N. 6
78. Jour. of the Reticuloendothelial Soc., Vol. 14, 1973
    Arch. Disease in Childhood, Vol. 49, 1974
79. Toxicology Letters, 2, 1978, p. 175
80. The Lancet, Sept. 17, 1977, p. 607

81. The Mer. Jour. Clin. Nutr., 30, Feb. 1977, p. 235
82. Z. Ernahrungswiss, 15, 1976, p. 387
83. Z. Ernahrungswiss, 16, 1977, p. 12
84. The Amer. Jour. Clin. Nutr., Oct. 30, 1977, p. 1680
85. Arch. Environ. Health, Vol. 28, 1974
86. Atherosclerosis, 24, 1976, p. 1
87. Annals of Thoracic Surgery, Vol. 24, N. 2, Aug. 1977
88. Cancer Res., 39, March 1979, p. 663
89. The Amer. Jour. Clin. Nutr., Vol. 30, N. 4, Apr. 1977, p. 641
90. New Zealand Medical Jour., Oct. 26, 1977
91. Human Nutrition, p. 123
92. Modern Medicine, Feb. 1, 1977
93. Indian Jour. Med. Res., 65, 6, Jun. 1977, p. 865
94. Jour. Human Nutr., 30, 1976, p. 333
95. Jour. Applied Nutr., Vol. 27, N. 2
96. Orthomolecular Psychiatry, Vol. 4, N. 4, 1975, p. 297
97. Physician's Handbook of Nutritional Science
98. Acta Vitamin. Enzymol., 1977, p. 31
99. The Lancet, Feb. 14, 1979, p. 403
100. Cancer Res., 39, Mar. 1979, p. 663
101. Chem.-Biol. Interactions, 9, 1974, p. 285
102. Internat. Jour. Vit. Nutr. Res., 47, 1977
     Acta. Vitamin. Enzymol., 31, 1977, p. 43

CHAPTER 14   VITAMIN D

1. Food Chemical News, Jan. 30, 1978, p. 17
2. Jour. Florida Med. Assoc., Vol. 66, N. 4
3. Archives Environ. Health, Vol. 32, N. 4, p. 160
4. J. C. E. & M., Vol. 42, N. 6, 1976
5. Jour. Prosthetic Dentistry, Vol. 41, N. 1, Jan. 1979
6. BMJ, Nov. 23, 1974
7. Ob. Gyn. News, Vol. 13, N. 16, Aug. 15, 1978, p. 4
8. Modern Medicine, Aug. 1, 1976, p. 89, and Aug. 15, 1978, p. 100
9. Jour. IAPM, Vol. 3, N. 2, p. 59
10. Jour. Amer. Ger. Society, Vol. 26, N. 7, p. 309
11. Modern Medicine, Aug. 1, 1976, p. 89
12. Federation Proceedings, Vol. 37, N. 3, Mar. 1, 1978, p. 333
13. Pediatric News, Vol. 13, N. 3, Mar. 1976, p. 32
    Jour. Human Nutr., 30, 1976, p. 333
14. Vitamin Manual
15. Hormones Metab. Res., 10, 1978, p. 553
16. New England Jour. Med., Vol. 298, N. 4, Jan. 26, 1978, p. 193

17. Arch. Environ. Health, Vol. 32, N. 4
    Nutr. Reviews, Vol. 36, N. 7, Jul. 1978
18. BMJ, Jan. 27, 1979, p. 221
19. Annals of Internal Med., 89, 1978, p. 965

CHAPTER 15   VITAMIN E

1. JAMA, Vol. 81, Sept. 15, 1923, p. 889
2. Medical Tribune, Vol. 17, N. 26, Aug. 18, 1976, p. 7
3. Federation Proceedings, Vol. 36, N. 3, Mar. 1, 1977, p. 1168
4. Jour. Clinical Investigation, Vol. 60, Jul. 1977, p. 233
5. Proc. Natl. Aca. Science USA, Vol. 71, N. 12, Dec. 1974, p. 4763
   Proc. Natl. Aca. Sci. USA, Vol. 74, N. 4, Apr. 1977, p. 1640
6. The Amer. Jour. Clin. Nutr., 29, May 1976, p. 569
7. Acta. Gerontol. Et Geriatrica Belgica, Vol. 3, N. 2, Apr. 1975
8. Proc. Fed. Nutr. Sci., Vol. 2, 1977, p. 347
9. Internat. Jour. Vit. Nutr. Res., 45(3), 1975, p. 251
10. Internat. Jour. Vit. Nutr. Res., 43, 1973, p. 283
11. The Amer. Jour. Clin. Nutr., 29, May 1976, p. 569
12. Jour. of Neurology and Exp. Neurology, 37(5), 1978
13. Clin. Res., 27(1), 1979
14. Jour. Applied Physiology, 45(6), 1978
15. The Med. Jour. of Australia, Jun. 11, 1977, p. 904
16. Jour. Amer. Geriatrics Society, Vol. 25, N. 9, p. 400
17. Dental Survey, Jul. 1976
18. Surgery, Gynecology, and Obstetrics, Vol. 86, N. 1, Jun. 1948
    Shute, W., Vitamin E For Ailing and Healthy Hearts, Pyramid, 1969
19. Nutrition Against Disease, p. 254
20. Internat. Jour. Vit. Nutr. Res., 48, 1978, p. 250
    Amer. Jour. Clin. Nutr., 29, May 1976, p. 569
21. JAMA, Vol. 144, N. 10, p. 831
22. Jour. Pediatrics, Vol. 90, N. 5, May 1977
23. The Amer. Jour. Clin. Nutr., 31, Jan. 1978, p. 100
    The Amer. Jour. Clin. Nutr., 30, Apr. 1977, p. 517
    FDA, US Dept. Commerce, PB-262-653, "Evaluations of Health Aspects of Tocopherols," p. 16
24. Internat. Jour. Vit. Nutr. Res., 47, 1977, p. 9
25. Japanese Heart Jour., Vol. 18, N. 3, 1977, p. 282
26. Same as N. 11
27. Medical World News, May 2, 1977, p. 22
28. New England Jour. Med., Vol. 289, N. 18, p. 979
29. Japanese Heart Journal, Vol. 18, N. 3, p. 277

30. Environ. Health Perspectives, Vol. 16, Aug. 1976
    Toxicology and Applied Pharmacol., 45(1), 1978, p. 247
    Agr. Food Chem., 20:481, 1972
31. Archives Environ. Health, Vol. 33, N. 6, p. 285
32. Same as N. 11
33. Internat. Jour. Radiation Biol. & Related Stud. Phys. Chem. & Med.,
    34(6), 1978
34. Brit. Jour. Radiology, 51, 1978, p. 822
35. Experientia, 54, 1978
36. The Amer. Jour. Clin. Nutr., Vol. 31, N. 4, Apr. 1978, p. 703
37. Internat. Jour. Vit. Nutr. Res., Vol. 46, N. 2, 1976
38. The Jour. of Nutr., Vol. 107, N. 3, p. 363
39. Reported at 68th meeting Amer. Assoc. Cancer Res. by W. McGuire
    (NCI)
40. Environ. Res., 17, 1978, p. 356
41. Experientia, 34(1), p. 110
42. Same as N. 7
43. Jour. of Pediatrics, Feb. 1977, Vol. 90, N. 2, p. 282
44. Pediatrics Res., Vol. 2, N. 4, 1977, p. 472
45. Medical World News, Oct. 3, 1977, p. 16
    Medical Tribune, Feb. 28, 1979, p. 1
    New England Jour. Med., Sept. 14, 1978
    Pediatric News, Vol. 2, N. 9, Sept. 1977, p. 46
    Nutr. Reviews, Vol. 37, N. 1, Jan. 1979
46. Medical World News, Oct. 3, 1977
    The Amer. Jour. Clin. Nutr., 29, May 1976
    Pediatrics, Vol. 63, N. 6, Jun. 1979
47. Pediatrics, Vol. 63, N. 6, Jun. 1979
48. Pediatric Res., 12(4), 1978, p. 525
49. Same as N. 11
50. Ob. Gyn. News, Vol. 2, N. 24, p. 17
51. Internat. Jour. Vit. Nutr. Res., 49, 1979
52. Jour. Amer. Geriatrics Soc., Vol. 26, N. 7, p. 328
53. Cutis, Vol. 21, Mar. 1978, p. 321
54. The Amer. Jour. Clin. Nutr., 31, Jan. 1978, p. 94
55. Same as N. 4
56. F. Amer. Soc. Exp. Biol., Apr. 1, 1979, Abstract N. 2540, 2016
57. Jour. Amer. Dental Assoc., Dec. 1975
58. Jour. Florida Med. Assoc., Vol. 66, N. 4, p. 408
59. Annals of Internal Medicine, Jan. 1979, p. 53
60. Israeli Jour. Medical Science, Jan. 1976
61. The Amer. Jour. of Clin. Nutr., 29, May 1976, p. 569

62. BioScience, Vol. 27, N. 7, Jul. 1977, p. 467
63. Acta Vitamin. Enzymol., Vol. 31, 1977, p. 143
64. Jour. Pediatrics, Feb. 1977
    Southern Medical Jour., Vol. 69, N. 10
65. F.A.S.E.B., 61st Annual Meeting, Apr. 1977
66. Internat. Jour. Vit. Nutr. Res., 43, 1973
67. New England Jour. Med., Vol. 289, N. 18
68. The Amer. Jour. Clin. Nutr., 31, May 1978, p. 831
69. FDA Publication SCOGS-36 Eval. Health Aspects of Tocopherols
70. JAMA, Vol. 230, N. 9, Dec. 2, 1974
71. Cutis, Vol. 21, Mar. 1978, p. 321
72. The Amer. Jour. Clin. Nutr., May 1978, p. 831
73. Cutis, Vol. 23, Jan. 1979, p. 49

CHAPTER 16   VITAMIN K

1. Journal of Dental Res., Vol. 56, 1977, p. 354
2. JAMA, Vol. 238, N. 1, July 4, 1977, p. 42
3. CMA Jour., Vol. 109, Nov. 3, 1973, p. 880
4. Jour. Human Nutr., 30, 1976, p. 333

CHAPTER 17   CALCIUM

1. Archives of Envirn. Health, Vol. 32, N. 4, Jul./Aug. 1977, p. 160
   Jour. Lab. Clin. Med., 91(3), Mar. 1978, p. 366
2. Science, Jan. 11, 1974
3. Environmental Res., 15, 1978, p. 175
4. Ob. Gyn. News, Vol. 13, N. 16, p. 4
5. Amer. Family Physician, Vol. 18, N. 4, Oct. 1978, p. 162
6. Annals of Internal Medicine, Vol. 89, 1978, p. 356
7. N.Y. State Jour. Medicine, Feb. 1975, p. 326
8. Ob. Gyn. News, Vol. 13, N. 16, p. 4
9. N.Y. State Jour. Med., Feb. 1975, p. 335
10. Cornell Vet., 62:32, 1972, p. 32
11. Jour. Prosthetic Dentistry, Vol. 41, N. 1, Jan. 1979
12. Same as N. 7
13. F.A.S.E.B. Proc., 1979, Abstr. N. 2870
    Annals of Internal Med., Vol. 87, N. 6, Dec. 1977, p. 649
    BMJ, Sept. 24, 1977, p. 789
14. Same as N. 7
15. Annals of Internal Med., Vol. 89, Sept. 1978, p. 356
16. Clinical Science and Molecular Med., 53, 1977, p. 579
17. Metabolism, Vol. 27, N. 12, Dec. 1978

18. Nutr. Rep. Internat., Vol. 117, N. 6, Jun. 1978
19. Nutr. Rep. Internat., Vol. 8, N. 2, Aug. 1973, p. 119
20. Same as N. 18
21. The Amer. Jour. Clin. Nutr., 30, Oct. 1977, p. 1603
22. Same as N. 10
23. Same as N. 21
24. Postgraduate Med., Vol. 60, N. 2, Aug. 1976, p. 75
25. Amer. Fam. Physician, Vol. 18, N. 4, Oct. 1978
26. Brit. Jour. Urology, 1978, 50, p. 459
27. Amer. F. P., Oct. 1979
    Jour. Clin. Endoc. Metab., Vol. 41, N. 6, 1975
    JAMA, Sept. 5, 1977, p. 1018
28. Same as N. 24
29. Same as N. 10
30. Pediatrics, Vol. 62, N. 5, Nov. 1978
31. Nutr. Rep. Internat., Vol. 18, N. 3, Sept. 1978, p. 313
    Jour. Amer. Dietetic Assoc., Vol. 70, N. 4, Apr. 1977, p. 368
32. The Amer. Jour. Clin. Nutr., 30, Oct. 1977, p. 603

CHAPTER 18 CHROMIUM

1. Jour. Applied Nutr., Vol. 30, N. 1&2, 1978, p. 14
    Trace Elements and Man, Schroeder, H. A.
 2. BMJ, Apr. 2, 1977, p. 905
 3. F.A.S.E.B., Apr. 1977, p. 1152
 4. Jour. Applied Nutr., Vol. 30, N. 1&2, 1978, p. 14
 5. Trends in Biochemistry, Dec. 1977, p. 277
 6. 11th Ann. Conf. Trace Elements in Environ. Health, Jun. 1977, p. 45
 7. Trace Elements and Man, Schroeder, H. A.
 8. F.A.S.E.B., Apr. 1977, Abstr. N. 4509, p. 1123
 9. Clin. Chem., 24(4), 1978, p. 541
10. Same as N. 7
11. Same as N. 7
12. Southern Medical Jour., 70(12), Dec. 1977, p. 1449
13. Medical World News, Vol. 15, N. 34, p. 33
14. Same as N. 5
15. Arch. Environ. Health, Vol. 28, Feb. 1974, p. 105

CHAPTER 19 COPPER

1. Food Product Development, May 1978
    New England Jour. Medicine, Aug. 11, 1977, p. 318
 2. F.A.S.E.B., Jun. 1977, p. 11
 3. F.A.S.E.B., Mar. 1978, Abstr. N. 324, p. 324

4. Jour. Applied Nutr., Vol. 27, N. 23, fall 1975
5. Orthomolecular Psychiatry, Vol. 4, N. 4, 1975, p. 297
6. JAMA, Vol. 241, N. 8, May 4, 1979
7. F.A.S.E.B., Apr. 1978, Abstr. N. 3585, p. 894
8. Medical World News, Feb. 20, 1978, p. 49

CHAPTER 20   FLUORINE

1. Environment, Vol. 16, N. 1, Jan./Feb. 1974, p. 12
2. Jour. Florida Med. Assoc., Vol. 66, N. 4
3. National Fluoridation News, Vol. 22, N. 1, Jan.-Mar. 1976
4. 172nd Amer. Chem. Soc. National Conf., N. 25, 1976
5. Jour. Florida Med. Assoc., Apr. 1979, p. 411
6. 172nd Amer. Chem. Soc. Annual Conf., N. 24, 1976
7. Same as N. 1
8. Fluoride, Vol. 12, N. 2, Apr. 1979, p. 55
9. Pediatrics, Vol. 49, N. 3, Mar. 1972
10. Fluoride, Vol. 11, N. 4, Oct. 1978, p. 163
11. Fluoride, Vol. 9, N. 1, Jan. 1976, p. 1
12. Fluoride, Vol. 12, N. 3, Jul. 1978, p. 111
13. Fluoride, Vol. 9, N. 1, Jan. 1976
14. Fluoride, Vol. 7, N. 1, Jan. 1974, p. 2
15. Environment, Vol. 16, N. 1
    Fluoride, Jan. 1974, p. 47
    Fluoride, Vol. 10, N. 1, Jan. 1977, p. 40
16. Same as N. 1
17. Ob. Gyn. News, Vol. 13, N. 16, p. 19
18. Postgraduate Medicine, Vol. 60, N. 2, Aug. 1976
19. Same as N. 14
20. Internat. Jour. Environmental Studies, Vol. 5, 1973, p. 141
21. Food Nutrition News, Vol. 33, N. 3, 1976

CHAPTER 21   IODINE

1. BMJ, Dec. 17, 1977, p. 1566
2. The Lancet, Apr. 24, 1976, p. 890
3. Jour. Nutr. Education, Vol. 8, N. 3, Jul.-Sept. 1976
4. Amer. Chem. Society News Service, Jun. 15, 1976
5. Jour. Nutr. Ed., Vol. 8, N. 3
    BMJ, Dec. 17, 1977, p. 1566
6. Arch. Dermatol., Vol. 112, Apr. 1976, p. 555
7. Amer. Jour. Clin. Nutr., 28, Jul. 1975, p. 712
    Pediatrics, Vol. 56, N. 1, Jul. 1975, p. 82

CHAPTER 22   IRON

1. Human Nutrition
2. New England Jour. Medicine, Sept. 8, 1977, p. 543
3. The Lancet, May 7, 1977, p. 1000
4. C & EN, Jan. 17, 1977, p. 35
5. Jour. Florida Med. Assoc., Apr. 1979, p. 413
6. The Amer. Jour. Clin. Nutr., 30, Jun. 1977, p. 910
7. Acta Med. Scand., Vol. 188, 1970, p. 361
8. F.A.S.E.B., Mar. 1978, Abstr. N. 1447, p. 487
   Jour. Amer. Dietetic Assoc., Oct. 1977
9. Jour. Pediatrics, Mar. 1976
10. Archives Environ. Health, Vol. 32, N. 4, 1977, p. 160
11. Environmental Health Perspectives, Dec. 1975, p. 77
12. F.A.S.E.B., Vol. 36, N. 5, Apr. 1977
    Nutr. Rep. Internatl., Vol. 16, N. 6, Dec. 1977, p. 769
13. Medical Jour. Australia, Sept. 27, 1974, p. 429
14. Jour. Amer. Dietetic Assoc., Vol. 70, N. 3, Mar. 1979, p. 260
15. Same as N. 14
16. Same as N. 2
17. Garry & Owen Univ. New Mexico Med. Sch. & U. Mich. Sch. Pub. Health
18. Fed. Proceedings, Vol. 36, N. 7, Jun. 1977, p. 2028
    Jour. Agric. Food Chem., Vol. 26, N. 1, 1978, p. 223
19. JAMA, Vol. 239, N. 19, May 12, 1978, p. 1999
20. Amer. Jour. Clin. Nutr., Feb. 1977
    Pediatrics, May 1975
21. The Jour. of Pediatrics, Vol. 91, Jul. 1977, p. 36

CHAPTER 23   MAGNESIUM

1. F.A.S.E.B. Proc., Vol. 35, N. 3, Mar. 1, 1976, Abstr. N. 1627
2. Clin. Ped., Vol. 13, N. 3, Mar. 1974, p. 263
3. The Amer. Jour. Medicine, Vol. 58, Jun. 1975
4. Jour. of Nutr., Vol. 107, N. 9, Sept. 1977, p. 1640
5. F.A.S.E.B. Proc., Vol. 36, N. 3, Mar. 1, 1977, Abstr. N. 4556
6. The Amer. Jour. of Med., Vol. 58, Jun. 1975, p. 841
   The Jour of Nervous and Mental Disease, Vol. 165, N. 6, p. 423
7. Clin. Pediatrics, Vol. 13, N. 3, Mar. 1974, p. 266
8. The Lancet, Feb. 5, 1977, p. 283
9. The Lancet, May 18, 1974, p. 963
10. The Amer. Jour. Clin. Nutr., 27:59, 1974
11. SA Med. Jour., Apr. 15, 1978, p. 591
12. The Amer. Jour. Clin. Nutr., 32, May 1979

13. New England Jour. Med., Apr. 14, 1977, p. 862
14. CMA Jour., Vol. 113, Aug. 9, 1975, p. 199
15. Same as N. 11
16. The Amer. Jour. Med., Vol. 58, Jun. 1975, p. 843
17. The Amer. Heart Jour., Vol. 93, N. 6, Jun. 1977, p. 679
18. Current Therapeutic Res., Vol. 4, N. 3, Mar. 1962, p. 98
19. Ob. Gyn. News, Vol. 12, N. 22, Nov. 15, 1977, p. 1
20. Internatl. Surgery, Vol. 61, N. 5, May 1976, p. 262
    The Aca. Jour. Chiropractic, Nov. 1974, p. 173
21. Same as N. 16
22. The Amer. Jour. Clin. Nutr., 14:342, 1964
23. Clin. Pediatrics, Mar. 1974, p. 263
24. Modern Medicine, Vol. 46, N. 5, Mar. 15, 1978
    The Amer. Jour. Med., Vol. 58, Jun. 1975, p. 837
25. The Jour. of Nervous and Mental Disease, Vol. 165, N. 6, p. 423
26. Clin. Pediatrics, Vol. 13, N. 3, p. 264
27. Same as N. 26
28. Jour. Amer. Dietetic Assoc., Vol. 70, N. 3, Mar. 1977

CHAPTER 24   MANGANESE

1. Brit. Jour. Nutr., Vol. 41, N. 2, 1979, p. 253
2. Arch. Environ. Health, Vol. 28, Feb. 1974, p. 109
3. Trace Ele. Metab. in Animals, Hoekstra, V. G.; Univ. Park Press, Baltimore, 1974, p. 51
4. Nutr. Rep. Internatl., Vol. 19, N. 2, Feb. 1979, p. 165
5. Fed. Proceedings, Vol. 35, N. 11, Sept. 1978
6. Same as N. 1
7. 12th Ann. Conf. Trace Elem. Environ. Health, Shamberger et al.
8. The Lancet, Dec. 29, 1962, p. 1348
9. JAMA, Vol. 238, N. 17, Oct. 24, 1977, p. 1805
10. Amer. Jour. Psychiatry, 133:1, Jan. 1976
11. Same as N. 1

CHAPTER 25   MOLYBDENUM

1. Underwood, E. J., Trace Elements in Animal and Human Nutr., Academic Press, N.Y. & London, 3rd Ed., 1971, p. 116
2. Human Nutrition
3. Arch. Environ. Health, Vol. 28, Feb. 1974, p. 109

CHAPTER 26   PHOSPHORUS

1. Drug Therapy, Aug. 1976, p. 114

2. Jour. Canadian Dietetic Assoc., Vol. 38, N. 2, Apr. 1977, p. 111
3. The Jour. of Nutr., Vol. 104, N. 9, Sept. 1974, p. 1195
4. The Jour. of Nutr., Vol. 107, N. 1, Jan. 1977, p. 42
5. Same as N. 4
6. Jour. of Food Science, Vol. 43, N. 5, 1978, p. 1473

CHAPTER 27 POTASSIUM

1. Medical Tribune, Vol. 18, N. 28, Sept. 14, 1977, p. 1
2. Internal Medicine, May 1, 1974, p. 10
3. JAMA, Vol. 237, N. 13, Mar. 28, 1977, p. 1305
4. Plant Foods Human Nutr., 23, 1/3, 1973, p. 3
5. Nutrition Reviews, Vol. 34, N. 8, Aug. 1976, p. 227
6. Medical World News, Apr. 17, 1978
7. The Amer. Jour. Clin. Nutr., 32, May 1979, p. 97
8. Internal Medicine, May 1, 1974, p. 10
   Modern Medicine, October 1, 1976, p. 97
9. Arch. Surgery, Vol. 112, Oct. 1977, p. 1165
10. Jour. Amer. Dietetic Assoc., Vol. 73, N. 1, Jul. 1978, p. 64
11. Internal Medicine News, Vol. 8, N. 2, Jan. 15, 1975, p. 5
12. The Lancet, Mar. 26, 1977, p. 704
13. Nutrition Reviews, Vol. 34, N. 8, Aug. 1976, p. 25
14. Internal Medicine, May 1, 1974, p. 10
15. Postgraduate Medicine, Vol. 57, N. 2, Feb. 1975, p. 123

CHAPTER 28 SELENIUM

1. Proc. Symposium on Selenium & Tellurium in the Environ.; Industrial
   Health Foundation, Inc., Pittsburgh, 1976, p. 129
   "Selenium in Biology," Frost, D., and Lish, P., Annual Review of
   Pharmacology, 15:259-84, 1975
2. Bioscience, Vol. 27, N. 7, p. 467
3. Jour. Amer. Dietetic Assoc., Vol. 66, Apr. 1975, p. 338
4. Same as N. 2
5. PSSTE (Symposium listed in N. 1), 1976, p. 129
6. Same as N. 2
7. Jour. Nutr. Science Vitaminol., 23:273, 1977
8. F.A.S.E.B. Proc., Vol. 36, N. 3, 1977, p. 1094
9. Pediatric News, Vol. 12, N. 7, Jul. 1978, p. 10
10. Same as N. 2
11. PSSTE, 1976, p. 253-67
12. "Selenium in Biology," Frost, D., and Lish, P. (See N. 1)
13. Same as N. 11
14. PSSTE, 1976, p. 293

15. PSSTE, 1976, p. 234
16. Same as N. 14
17. Same as N. 3
18. Arch. Environ. Health, Vol. 28, Feb. 1974
19. JAMA, Vol. 237, N. 26, p. 2843
20. Same as N. 12
21. Bioinorganic Chemistry, 8:303, 1978

CHAPTER 29   SILICON

1. Federation Proc., Vol. 33, N. 6, Jun. 1974, p. 1758
   The Amer. Jour. of Clin. Nutr., 27, May 1974, p. 515
   Nutr. Reviews, Vol. 33, N. 9, Sept. 1975, p. 257
   Schwarz, K., Nature, 239:333
2. Federation Proc., Vol. 33, N. 6, Jun. 1974, p. 1758
3. The Amer. Jour. Surgery, Vol. 119, May 1970, p. 560
4. Military Medicine, Vol. 130, N. 11, Nov. 1965
5. The Lancet, Feb. 26, 1977, p. 454
6. Angiology, May 1973
7. The Amer. Jour Clin. Nutr., 27, May 1974, p. 515

CHAPTER 31   ZINC

1. Pediatrics, Vol. 62, N. 3, Sept. 1978, p. 408
2. Medical Clinics of North America, Vol. 60, Jul. 1976, p. 675
3. Crit. Rev. in Clin. Lab. Sciences, Vol. 8, N. 1, Sept. 1977, p. 1
   Food Nutr. News, Vol. 33, N. 3, 1976, p. 96
   Jour. of Nutr., Vol. 107, N. 5, May 1977, p. 855
   Nutr. Rep. Internat., Vol. 16, N. 3, Sept. 1977, p. 267
   Jour. of Nutr., Vol. 107, N. 10, Oct. 1977, p. 1889
4. Same as N. 1
5. Jour. Human Nutr., Vol. 32, N. 2, 1978, p. 99
6. Western Jour. Med., Vol. 130, N. 2, Feb. 1979, p. 133
7. Same as N. 5
8. European Jour. Pharmacol., Vol. 48, 1978, p. 97
9. Trace Substances in Environ. Health, Vol. 7, 1973, Flynn, Strain, Pories, & Hill, Univ. Mo., Columbia, p. 271
10. The Amer. Jour. Clin. Nutr., Vol. 30, N. 4, Apr. 1977, p. 612
11. Medical World News, Feb. 7, 1977, p. 57
12. Tennican, P.O. Univ. Arizona Health Sciences Center, Tucson
13. Symposium on Clin. Applications of Zinc Metab., Pories & Strain, Cleveland Met. Gen. Hospital, Case Western Reserve Univ. Sch. of Med.
14. Gynecology Oncology, 4, 1976, p. 324
15. Southern Med. Jour., Vol. 70, N. 5, May 1977, p. 559

16. Brit. Jour. Dermatol., Vol. 96, 1977, p. 283
17. Fed. Proceedings, Vol. 37, N. 3, Mar. 1978, p. 253, Abstr. N. 215
18. Brit. Jour Dermatol., Vol. 97, 1977, p. 679
19. The Lancet, Sept. 11, 1976, p. 539
20. Brit. Heart Jour., 38, 1976, p. 1339
21. Henzel, Holtmann, Katzer, Deweese, Licht: Dept. Surgery, Univ. Mo. Med. Center 1968—Proc. 2nd Annual Conf. Trace Sub. Environ. Health
22. JAMA, Vol. 235, N. 22, May 31, 1976
23. Bush; Cook Co. Hospital—AMA Annual Meeting, Chicago, 1974
24. The Lancet, Oct. 29, 1977, p. 895
25. Sexual Medicine Today, Nov. 1978
26. Same as N. 6
27. Proc. Soc. Exp. Biol. and Med., 154, 1977, p. 146
28. Fed Proceedings, N. 1018, 1978, p. 405
29. Fed. Proc., 1977, p. 1152, N. 4656, and p. 1685, N. 5
30. Food Nutr. News, Vol. 33, N. 3, 1976
31. Same as N. 13, plus: Med. Clin. North Amer., Vol. 60, N. 4, Jul. 1976
    Western Journal of Med., Vol. 130, N. 2, Feb. 1979, p. 133
    Postgraduate Medical Jour., 53, Mar. 1977, p. 143
32. Nutr. Reviews, Vol. 37, N. 3, Mar. 1979, p. 76
33. Fed. Proceedings, Vol. 35, N. 11, Sept. 1978, N. 2271
    Jour. Human Nutr., 32, 1978, p. 99
34. Same as N. 6
35. Medical World News, Aug. 4, 1972, p. 62
36. Same as N. 6
37. JAMA, Vol. 241, N. 18, May 4, 1979, p. 1916
38. Jour. Amer. Dietetic Assoc., Vol. 70, N. 3, Mar. 1977, p. 260
39. Same as N. 35
40. Western Jour. Med., Vol. 130, N. 2, Feb. 1979, p. 133
    Fed. Proc., Mar. 1979, Abstr. N. 1685, 1694
    Fed. Proc., Vol. 37, N. 3, 1978, Abstr. N. 216
41. Clin. Res., 23, 1975, p. 222A
42. Clin. Res., 26, 1978, p. 701A
43. Pediatrics, Vol. 62, N. 3, Sept. 1978, p. 408
    Jour. of Nutr., Vol. 107, N. 2, p. 2219
44. Arch. Environ. Health, Vol. 28, Feb. 1974, p. 105
45. Food Nutr. News, Vol. 33, N. 3, 1970, p. 98
46. Same as N. 6
47. Same as N. 6

CHAPTER 32 OTHER MINERALS

1. Schwarz, Klaus, "New Essential Trace Elements: Progress Report and Outlook," Trace Element Metab. in Animals, 2, Hoekstra, Suttie, Ganther, Mertz, Univ. Park Press, 1974, pp. 335-78

CHAPTER 33   BIOFLAVONOIDS

1. Qual. Plant Foods Hum. Nutr., 23, 1/3, 1973, p. 119
   Clin. Chem., 17, 1971, p. 433
2. Internatl. Jour. Vit. Nutr. Res., 43, 1973, p. 494
   Clin. Chemistry, Vol. 17, N. 5, 1971
3. Proc. Soc. Exp. Biol. & Med., 95, 1957, p. 660
4. Sokoloff, Martin, Saelhof—20th Internatl. Congress of Physiology, Brussels, Belgium 1956
5. Medical World News, Oct. 12, 1973
6. Family Practice News, Apr. 15, 1973
   Rev. Fr. Gynecol. & Obstet., Vol. 68, 1973, p. 345
7. Chicago Med., Mar. 7, 1964
8. Geriatrics, Vol. 8, N. 2, 1953
9. Rutin & Related Flav., Griffith, Krewson, Mack Pub. Co., 1955
10. Oral Surgery, Vol. 45, N. 1, Jun. 1978
11. Same as N. 9

CHAPTER 34   THE OUTLAW VITAMINS

1. New York Magazine, March 13, 1978
2. N.Y. State Jour. of Med., Sept. 1978
3. Orthomolecular Psychiatry, Vol. 4, N. 2, 1975
4. Wall Street Journal, Apr. 4, 1978
5. New England Jour. Med., Vol. 299, N. 10, 1978, p. 549
6. Annals of Internal Med., Vol. 89, N. 3, Sept. 1978
7. Same as N. 6
8. Soc. Science and Med., Vol. 12, 1978, p. 31
9. Medical World News, Feb. 2, 1973
   Medical Tribune, Sept. 26, 1973
   Chem. & Eng. News, Dec. 3, 1973
   Life Sciences, Vol. 15, p. 1
10. California Medicine, Jan. 1949 and Jan. 1956
11. Jour. Amer. Medical Women's Assoc., Vol. 18, N. 6
    JAMA, July 23, 1973
    Postgraduate Medical Jour., Vol. 51, Jun. 1975, p. 366

Index

Abortions, spontaneous, 86–87
Absorption of nutrients, and zinc, 258
Acetaldehyde toxicity, 74
Acetaminophen, 148, 174
Acetylcholine, 115–16
Achlorhydria, 104
Acne, 261
  and fluorine, 216
  and iodine, 219
  premenstrual, 69–70
Acrodermatitis enteropathica, 258–65
Addiction to raw eggs and wine, 100–101
Adrenal glands, 21–22, 45–46, 101–102, 106–10, 126–27, 259, 275
Adriamycin, 174–75
Aggregation, blood cell, 274–76
  platelet, 170–71
Aging, 123, 279–81
  and pyridoxine, 76
  and selenium, 246
  and silicon, 252–53
  and vitamin E, 165–66, 168–69
Air pollution, 173
Albanese, Dr. Anthony, 194–96
Alcohol, 36–37, 41–42, 52, 89, 147, 264
Alcoholism, 103, 232, 239, 243, 246, 279–81
Alertness, 147
Allergic response, 145

Allergies, 111, 275, 279
  to fluoride, 216
Alpha tocopherol, 183
Alveolar bone loss, 197–98
Alveolar ridge, 158–59
Alzheimer's Disease, 115–17
Amino acids, 4, 62–63, 126, 149
Aminopterin, 89
Aminosalicylic acid, 243
Ammonium chloride, 243
Amnesia, 37
Amphoterin, 243
Amygdalin, 281
Anderson, Dr. Terence, 135
Anemia, 101
  and copper, 210
  and folate, 80
  hemolytic, 175
  and iron, 222–24
  macrocytic, 87–88
  megaloblastic, 92–93
  pernicious, 92–94
  and riboflavin, 47
  and thiamine, 37–38
  and vitamin A, 21–22
Anesthesia, 232
Anesthetic drugs, 259
Angina, 170, 172, 248, 254, 279
Anorexia, 243
Antacids, 199, 239

315

Antibiotics, 50, 104, 137, 185, 199
Antibodies, 107, 137
Anticoagulant drugs, 182
Anticonvulsants, 89, 160, 199
Antidepressant drugs, 232
Antimony, 124
Antioxidants, 21, 124, 127, 164–66, 245–46, 257
Anxiety, 53, 117, 244, 279
Aorta, 216
Apathy, 81–82
Apnea, 103, 228
Appetite, 36, 53, 228, 258
Arrhythmia, cardiac, 229–30, 244
Arsenic, 124
Arteries and fluorine, 216
Arteriosclerosis and vitamin D, 161
Arthritis, 57–58, 67–68, 110, 138, 145–46, 157, 177, 216, 261–62, 275
Ascorbic acid. *See* vitamin C
Aspirin, 151
Atherosclerosis, 84–85, 131–34, 204–206
Athletic performance, 43, 47–48, 103
ATP-ADP, 227
Autism, 72, 279–81
Autoimmune disease, 177–78
Avidin, 101, 104

"Baby Blues," 87–88
Barbiturates, 89
    and vitamin C, 151
    and vitamin K, 186
Beriberi, 36, 41
Beta tocopherol, 183
Bilirubin lights and riboflavin, 49
Bioflavonoids, 273–77, 289
Biotin, 100–104, 123
    and pantothenate, 113
Birth canal, narrowing, 157
Birth defects, 46, 214
Bishop, Dr. Katherine, 163
Bladder tumors, 74
Bleeding
    and iron, 222–24
    and vitamin E, 182
    and vitamin K, 185
Bleeding gums, 196
Blood, 238
    clotting, 191, 196, 234, 283
    oxygenation, 279
Blood platelets, 93
Blood pressure, 255–56
    and copper, 210

    and pantothenate, 106
    and vitamin C, 132
    and vitamin E, 172
Blood sugar, 146
Blood vessels, 252–56
    and niacin, 51–52, 56–57
Bone marrow and folate, 79
Bones, 126–27, 238, 252
    and calcium, 190–200
    and copper, 209
    and fluoride, 216
    and magnesium, 228
    and vitamin D, 155–62
    and vitamin K, 184–85
Brain, 252
    dysfunction, 279
    and fluorine, 216
    and folate, 81
    and vitamin E, 167
Breast cysts, 176–77
Breastfeeding, 102
Breast milk, 191, 258
Breath-holding spells, 72
Bronchopulmonary dysplasia, 175
Burning sensations, 68
Burns, 265
    eye, 130
    and zinc, 260

Cadmium, 148, 192, 213, 223, 249, 264, 267, 270
Calamine, 260
Calcium, 8, 160, 189–200
    and magnesium, 227–29, 232
    and phosphorus, 238–40
    and vitamin C, 149
    and vitamin D, 155–60
Cameron, Dr. Ewan, 138–45, 153
CAMP, 146
Campbell, Dr. Allan, 141
Cancer, 265
    breast, 176–77
    and choline, 118–19
    and folate, 90
    and inositol, 121
    and iodine, 218–19
    and laetrile, 281–82
    and PABA, 123
    and pyridoxine, 73–74
    and riboflavin, 48
    and selenium, 245, 248–49
    and thiamine, 39
    and vitamin A, 26–28

and vitamin C, 136–46
Capillaries
    and bioflavonoids, 273–77
    and vitamin C, 126, 134–35
Carbenicillin, 243
Carbenoxolone, 243
Carbohydrate metabolism, 65, 238, 246
    and biotin, 101
    and chromium, 204, 206–207
    and pantothenate, 106
    and pyridoxine, 62
    and riboflavin, 45
    and thiamine, 35–36
Carbohydrates, 5
Carbon dioxide exchange, 257
Carcinogens, 144
Cardiac irregularities, 241
Carpal tunnel syndrome, 68–69
Cartilage, 126, 155, 234, 252
Cataracts, 46, 135
Cell, 4, 6, 44, 51, 62, 79–80, 106, 126,
    146, 164–66, 181, 209, 221–22, 227,
    241–42, 245–47, 255–58, 270, 279
    membranes, 165–66, 173–74, 247
Central nervous system, 128
Cesarean section and BPD, 175
Charley horses, 68
Chelating agents, 267
Cheney, Dr. Garnett, 284
Children
    diabetic, 66
    and pyridoxine, 63, 70–72, 76
    and riboflavin, 49
Chlorine, 269
Cholesterol, 102
    and adrenal gland, 106–107
    and calcium, 196–97
    and chromium, 202, 205
    and copper, 210
    and folate, 84–85
    and manganese, 235
    and niacin, 51–52, 56–57
    and pyridoxine, 64
    and vitamin C, 132–33, 135
    and vitamin D, 156
    and vitamin E, 171
Cholestyramine, 98
Choline, 114–19
Chondroitin sulfate, 254
Chope, Dr. Harold, 3
Chromium, 201–8, 235
    and vitamin C, 149
Chromosomes, 270

damage by fluoride, 214
Chronic liver disease, 43
Circulatory disease, 3
Cirrhosis, 232, 265
Clomiphene, 128
Clots, blood, 133–34, 170–71
Clotting disorders, 246
Clumping of blood cells, 274–75
Coagulation, blood, 184–85
Cobalamin, 91–99
    and choline, 114
    and folate, 80
    and thiamine, 42
    vegetable sources of, 99
Cobalt, 92
Coenzyme A, 106, 111
Coffee and thiamine, 42
Colchicine, 98
Colds and vitamin C, 135–37, 147
Cold sores, 131, 276
Cold stress, 109–10, 129, 228
Colic, 153
Colitis, ulcerative, 110–11
Collagen, 63, 73, 126–27, 138, 209
Color perception, 93
Concentration
    and riboflavin, 47
    and thiamine, 36
    and vitamin C, 147
Confusion, 83, 244
Congestive heart failure, 49, 182, 232
Connective tissue, 126, 252, 257
Continuum, 2, 37, 57, 78, 81, 101
Convulsions, 64, 107
    and copper, 210
    in infants, 62
    and magnesium, 228–29
    and pyridoxine, 70–71, 74, 76
Copper, 209–11, 249, 257–58
    and vitamin C, 151
Corn and pellagra, 58–60
Corneal opacities, 202
corpus luteum, 126
Corticosteroids, 151, 160, 243, 267
Cortisone, 25
Cott, Dr. Allan, 280
Cow's milk and copper, 209–10
Cramps
    leg, 68
    muscular, 255
Cretinism, 218
CSA, 254
Cyanide, 281

Cyanocobalamin, 91
Cycloserine, 89
Cystic fibrosis, 165, 178
Cysts, breast, 176–77
Cytochrome, 222

Death, sudden, 101
DeBakey, Dr. Michael E., 171
decongestants, 72
Deficiency, 6–9
    local, 286–87
    of vitamin C, 152
Dehydration, 267
Delirium, 81–82
Delta tocopherols, 183
Dementia, 81–82
    and niacin, 53
    and vitamin C, 146
Demineralization of bone, 158–59
Dependency, pyridoxine, 64
Depression, 81–82, 101, 117, 258
    and cobalamin, 94
    and folate, 80
    and niacin, 53
post-partum, 87–88
    premenstrual, 69–70
    and pyridoxine, 65, 67, 77
    and riboflavin, 46–47
    and thiamine, 36
    and vitamin C, 127
Dermatitis, 53, 64, 100–102, 235, 258–
        59, 279
    and fluorine, 216
    seborrheic, 46
Detoxification, 147–49, 245, 249, 279
Diabetes, 60, 65, 234–35, 265, 275, 279–
        81
    and BPD, 175
    and chromium, 202–208
    and inositol, 120
    and magnesium, 232
    and pyridoxine, 66–67
    and vitamin C, 134–35, 146
    and vitamin E, 182
Diabetic children and riboflavin, 49
Diabetic ketoacidosis, 239
Dialysis, kidney, and copper, 210
Diarrhea, 53, 80, 94, 210, 239, 244
Diet, general guidelines, 13
Digestive disorders, 127
Digestive tract disease and vitamin C, 3
Digitalis, 230
Diphenylhydantoin, 89

Discoid lupus erythematosus, 178
Diuresis and vitamin C, 153
Diuretics, 243, 267
    and calcium, 199
Dizziness, 267
    and magnesium, 228
Down's syndrome, 265
Drowsiness, 80, 94
    and magnesium, 232
Drugs
    addiction, 279–81
    interfere with nutrients, 14
    and selenium, 246
    vs. vitamins, 286
Dwarfism, 259, 265

Eclampsia of pregnancy, 231
Edema, leg, 276
EDTA and iron, 225
Egg white injury, 101
Elastin and copper, 209
Elderly
    and biotin, 103
    and vitamin C, 150
Ellis, Dr. John M., 68–69
Emaciation, 127
Embryonic development, 252
Emetic, zinc, 267–68
Emotional instability, 53
Energy
    and B vitamins, 7
    and magnesium, 231
    metabolism, 279
    and pantothenate, 107
    production, 237
    and pyridoxine, 62
    and riboflavin, 45–46
    and thiamine, 41
    transfer, 245
Enteritis, 107
Epilepsy, 235
Epileptics and folate, 90
Epinephrine, 275
Epithelial tissues and vitamin A, 20
Essential fatty acids, 5–6
Estrogen, 89, 98
    and bone loss, 195–96
    and vitamin C, 151
    and vitamin E, 181–82
Evans, Dr. Herbert, 163
Excretion and iron, 222
Exercise, 131, 243–44
    and osteoporosis, 158–59, 195–96

and vitamin E, 168
Exercise tolerance, 254
Eyes
    inflamed, and riboflavin, 46
    and vitamin A, 22–23

Faddism, 15–16, 58
"Failure to thrive" syndrome, 49
Fascuculation, 228
Fast food meals, 30
Fat, 5–6, 118, 246
    and calcium, 199
    and niacin, 52
    metabolism, 45, 62, 64, 106, 202, 234,
        238
    mobilization, 52
Fatigue, 36–37, 47, 53, 57, 82–83, 108,
        127, 147, 231, 279–81
Fat-soluble vitamins, 289–90
Fatty acids, 101, 164–65, 167, 171, 173–
        74, 180–81, 237
Fertility, 69–70, 128
Fever and thiamine, 42
Fiber, interference with nutrients, 199,
        290
Fibrillation, ventricular, 230, 241
Fibrinolytic activity and vitamin C, 133
Fibrotic skin diseases, 123
Fight or flight response, 21
Fingernails and folate, 79
Fingers, swollen, 68
Flatulence and vitamin C, 153
Fluoridation, 212–17
Fluoride as a pollutant, 214
Fluorine, 212–17, 270
Fluorosis, 215–16
Folacin. See folate
Folate, 78–90
    and cobalamin, 92–94
    and gray hair, 123
    and pantothenate, 113
    and vitamin C, 126
Folic acid. See folate
Fracture risk, 195
Fractures and vitamin D, 158–59
Friedreich's Ataxia, 115–17
Friendliness and vitamin C, 147
Frostbite, 276
Fungus infection, 24

G6PD deficiency, 179
Gamma tocopherol, 183
Gangrene, 170, 279–81

Garden of Eden, nutritional, 125
Gastric surgery, 160
Gastrointestinal tract and niacin, 52–53
Genetic defects, 179–80
Gestational diabetes, 66
Gilles de la Tourette's Disease, 115–17
Gingivitis, 194
Glaucoma, 279–81
Glucagon, 243
Glucose, 5
    intravenous, 239
Glucose tolerance, 65–66, 234–35, 243
    and chromium, 202–208
    and folate, 83–84
Glucose tolerance factor (GTF), 202–
        208
Glutathione peroxidase, 246–47, 249
Glycogen, 5
Goiter, 218–20
Gonads and vitamin E, 166
Gout, 60
Gray hair, 107–108, 123
Growth, impaired, 127, 147, 202, 251
Gums, inflammation of, 63, 85–86, 179

Hair, 127, 235
    and biotin, 101
    and folate, 79
    and iron, 222
    and silicon, 252
Hallucinations, 53, 228
Haloperidol, 115
Hard water and heart disease, 196–97,
        230
Hartnup's Disease, 59
HDLs and vitamin C, 133
Headaches, 255
    and fluorine, 216
    and iron, 222
    and magnesium, 231
    and niacin, 53
Healing, 3, 25, 111, 127–31, 148, 169,
        252–53, 258, 260–61
Heart disease, 235, 264, 279–81
    and bioflavonoids, 274–76
    and biotin, 101
    and calcium, 196–97
    and choline, 118
    and copper, 210
    and chromium, 204–206
    and fluoride, 216
    and folate, 84–85
    and magnesium, 229–30

and niacin, 56–58
and potassium, 242–43
and pyridoxine, 72–73
and selenium, 245, 247–48
and silicon, 253–54
and vitamin C, 131–34
and vitamin E, 169–72
and zinc, 262
Heat stress and vitamin C, 129
Hemochromatosis, 225
Hemoglobin, 4, 221–22
  synthesis, 237
Hemorrhaging, 127
  and fluorine, 215–16
Hemorrhoids, 276
Heparin, 199
Hepatitis, 137, 265
Herniated disc, 157
Herpes, 96, 131, 137, 260, 276
Hesperidin, 273
High blood pressure, 60, 134, 148, 241–
    45, 275–76, 279–81
  and vitamin E, 182
High protein diet, 198–99, 267
Hives and fluorine, 216
Hodgkin's Disease, 73
Hoffer, Dr. Abram, 55
Hormone regulation, 279
Hospital malnutrition, 89
Hot flashes, 276
Housewife syndrome, 231
Huntington's Disease, 115–17
Hyaluronidase, 138–39, 142
Hydrazine, 74–75
Hydroperoxide, 246
Hyperactivity, 71
Hyperkeratinization, 22
Hyperparathyroidism, 239
Hyperthyroidism, 42, 150, 167, 182, 219,
    239
Hypnotic drugs, 160
Hypochondria, 47, 117, 127
Hypoglycemia, 83–84, 203
Hysteria, 127
  and riboflavin, 47
  vitamin, 278–83

Immune response, 80, 102, 107, 146,
    148, 258–60, 279–80
  and cancer, 139–40
  and choline, 114
  and cobalamin, 96
  and folate, 79

and iron, 222
and pyridoxine, 64, 74
and riboflavin, 48
and vitamin A, 24, 27–28
and vitamin C, 136, 146
and vitamin E, 168–69, 177–78
Impotence, 263–64
Incoordination, muscular, 267
Indians, North American, 60
Indigestion, 80
Indomethacin, 67
Infant formulas, 244, 265
Infants
  convulsions, 62
  and vitamin E, 175–76
Infections, 265, 275
  and folate, 80, 89
  respiratory, 108
  rickettsial, 123
  and thiamine, 38
  and vitamin A, 23–24
  and vitamin C, 135–37
  and zinc, 259–61
Infertility, 247
Inflammation, oral, 46–47, 53, 64, 80,
    94
Inflammatory disease, 179, 245, 265
Injury and iron, 222
Inositol, 120–21
Insecticides, 148
Insomnia, 53, 81–82, 101, 117, 210, 231
Insulin, 67, 201–202, 204, 234, 243
Interferon, 136–37
Intermittent claudication, 171–72
Intestinal distress, 216, 239
Intravenous feeding, 42, 89
Intrinsic factor, 92, 97
Iodide, 218–20
Iron, 8, 221–26
  and cobalamin, 93
  and molybdenum, 237
  and riboflavin, 47
  and vitamin C, 148–49, 223, 225
  and vitamin E, 175, 181
Iron supplements mistakenly given, 22
Irritability, 53, 57, 71, 80–82, 94, 108,
    157, 228, 241
Isoniazid, 71, 74, 89
Itching, 60
IUD, 276

Jaundice, neonatal, 49, 246
Jaw bone, 193

Joint swelling and fluorine, 216

Kaufman, Dr. William, 57–58
Keratinous tissue, 245
Kidneys, 159–61, 216, 228
Klevay, Dr. Leslie, 210
Kryptopyrrole (KP), 70

Lactation, 41, 77
Lactic acid, 35
Lactose, 200
Laetrile. *See* vitamin B$_{17}$
Lassitude, 101–102, 231
Laxative effects of magnesium, 232
Laxatives and nutrient loss, 160, 181,
    199, 243
LDLs, 133
Lead, 249, 270
    and calcium, 192
    and iron, 223
    and vitamin C, 148
    and zinc, 264
Lead poisoning, 164, 174
Learning disorders, 46, 223
Lecithin, 119, 121
Leg ulcers, 169–70
Leigh's Disease, 37
Leiner's Disease, 102
Lethargy, 46–47, 108, 228, 232, 267
Leukemia, 141, 265
Leukocytes and folate, 79, 96, 140
Levodopa, 77
Libido, 95–96
Licorice, 243
Ligaments, 252
Library of Congress, 214
Lind, James, 128, 134
Liver, 52, 64, 107, 114, 118–19, 121, 148,
    216, 252
Liver disease, 42, 60, 246–47, 279
Longevity, 3, 111–12, 202, 242
Loose teeth, 196
Loss of appetite, 101–102, 108
Low back pain, 131, 231
Low blood pressure, 244
Low blood sugar, 83–84
Low protein diet, 112–13, 207
Low-salt diet, 112–13
Lungs, 216, 247, 252
Lupus erythematosus, 123, 183
Lymphocytes and folate, 80, 136–37, 140

Macrocytic anemia, 87–88

Macronutrients, 4
Macrophages, 24, 136
Magnesium, 227–33, 257–58
    and copper, 210
Malabsorption, 186, 239, 265
Malnutrition
    in hospital, 89, 98, 185, 266
    protein-calorie, 203
Manganese, 70, 210, 234–36, 257–58
Manic depression, 115–17, 146–47
"Mauve factor," 70
Measles, 137
Megaloblastic anemia, 79–80
Melanin, 209
Memory, 36, 41, 81–82, 116–17
Meningitis, 137
Menke's kinky hair syndrome, 210
Menopausal arthritis, 68–69
Menopausal drugs, 151, 181
Menopause, 195, 276
Menorrhagia, 25–26, 276
Menstrual disorders, 275–77
Menstrual symptoms, 69–70
Menstruation and iron, 222–24
Mental disorientation, 241
Mental health, 94–96, 146
Mental illness, 54–55, 58, 70, 81
Mental retardation, 63–64, 81–82
Mercury, 175, 249
Metabolism and phosphorus, 238
Metformin, 98
Methionine and choline, 114
Methotrexate, 89, 98
Metrorrhagia, 276
Micronutrients, definition, 6
Milk and heart disease, 84–85
Miscarriage and fluorine, 214
Molybdenum, 237
Morning sickness, 66
Morphea, 178
Mother's milk and biotin, 102, 200, 226
Motivation, 228
Motor development, retarded, 87
Mottling, tooth, 215
Mouth ulcers, 216
Mucopolysaccharides, 252
Mucous membranes, 20, 53, 79
Multiple sclerosis, 38–39
Mumps, 137
Muscles, 127, 167, 191, 227, 238, 252
    coordination, 234
    cramps, 168
    degeneration, 247

pain, 101
tremors, 228
weakness, 127, 182, 241
Muscular dystrophy, 167, 178
Myoglobin, 222

Nausea, 60, 66, 101–102, 111, 216, 235
Neomycin, 98
Nerve conduction, 120, 227–29, 241
Nerve degeneration, 64
Nervousness, 36, 231
Nervous system, 3, 40, 52–53, 62, 79–
    80, 86–87, 92–94, 101–102, 115–18,
    146, 167, 191–93, 209, 238
Neuralgia, 279
Neurasthenia, 36
Neuritis, 279
Neurological deterioration, 93–94, 115–
    17, 127
Neuromuscular disorders, 64, 101
Neuropathy
    diabetic, 66–67
    optic, 93
Neurosis, 41
Neurotransmitters, 36, 146
Newborns and vitamin K, 185
Niacin, 3, 51–60, 114
    and pyridoxine, 62, 70, 77
Niacinamide. See niacin
Niacin flush, 52, 59–60
Nickel, 270
Nicotinic acid. See niacin
Night blindness, 20–21, 23
Nitrates, 148–49
Nitrites, 144, 148–49
Nitroglycerin, 84, 172
Nitrosamines, 148–49
Nitrous oxide, 172
Nosebleeds, 275
Nucleic acids, 78–79, 92, 202, 234, 245,
    257
Numbness, 68, 80, 94, 108

Obsessive-compulsive behavior, 55
Older women and thiamine, 42
Optimum health, 2–4, 14, 78, 151, 257,
    291
Oral contraceptives, 98, 267, 276
    and folate, 86, 89
    and pyridoxine, 64–65, 67, 75
    and riboflavin, 49–50
    and thiamine, 42
    and vitamin C, 151

and vitamin E, 177, 181–82
Orthomolecular psychiatry, 54, 70, 146–
    47
Osteitis, 160
Osteomalacia, 156–58
    and fluorine, 216
Osteoporosis, 158–59, 192–94, 210, 216,
    239
Oster, Dr. Kurt, 84–85
Oxalate excretion, 153
Oxygen, 4
Ozone, 123–24, 173

PABA, 122–24
Paget's Disease, 145
Pain, 231
    abdominal, 36, 267
    chest, 36
    muscular, and fluoride, 216
Pallor, 80, 94, 222
Pancreas and fluorine, 216
Pancreatic function, 245
Pancreatitis, 232
Pangamate. See vitamin B_{15}
Pangamic acid. See vitamin B_{15}
Pantothenate, 105–13
Pantothenic acid. See pantothenate
Para-aminobenzoic acid. See PABA
Paracetamol, 148, 174
Paralysis, 68, 241
Paranoia, 95–96, 117
Parkinsonism, 77, 236
Pauling, Linus, 135, 139–45
PCBs, 30, 148
Pellagra, 52, 56–59
Pemphigus, 123
Penicillin, 243
Pentamidine, 89
Pentane, 168
Periodontal disease, 179, 193, 222
Pernicious anemia, 80
Personality, 146
Peyronie's Disease, 123
Phagocytosis, 140
Phenformin, 98
Phenobarbitone, 89
Phenothiazine, 89, 115
Phenytoin, 89
PHI (physiological hyaluronidase
    inhibitor), 138–39, 142
Phosphate additives, 239–40
Phosphorus, 8, 238–40, 253
    and calcium, 199–200

and magnesium, 232
in vegetarians, 160
and vitamin D, 155-60
Pica, 222
"Pins and needles," 36
Pituitary gland, 126, 156
Pituitary, thyroid, 167
Plaques, 202
Plasmologen, 85
Platelet aggregation, 133-34
Platelet function, 196
Pneumonia, 24, 137
Poliomyelitis virus, 137
Polymyositis, 178
Polyneuropathy, 81-82
Polyps, rectal, 143-44
Porphyria cutanea tarda, 178
Potassium, 241-44, 256
and magnesium, 228, 231
time-release, 244
Potassium chloride, 98
Potency, 263-64
Pregnancy, 28-29, 41, 46-47, 63-64, 66,
73, 75-76, 86-89, 96-97, 103-104,
107-108, 112-13, 128-29, 191, 199,
223-24, 231, 234-35, 245, 258, 265,
276
depression in, 65
Premature infants, 175-76, 247
Premenstrual depression, 65
Presenile dementia, 115-17
Prickly heat, 131
Primidone, 89
Processed foods, 199-200, 239-40
Prolactin and pyridoxine, 70
Prostaglandins, 166, 246
Prostate, 259-60, 263
Protein, 4-5
metabolism, 45, 106, 202, 238
synthesis, 36, 101, 234, 257, 279
Psoriasis, 85
Psychiatric disturbances, 46-47, 258
Psychosis, 53, 95-96, 210, 228
post-partum, 87-88
Puberty, 166
Purgatives, 243
Pyridoxine, 61-77
and heart disease, 205
and niacin, 59
and riboflavin, 44
and thiamine, 42
Pyrimethamine, 89
Pyruvic acid, 35

Quercetin, 273
Quick, Dr. Armand J., 283-84

Rabies, 137
Radiation, 111, 138, 173-74
Radiation therapy, 138, 140-41
Radioactive iodine, 219
Raynaud's Phenomenon, 178
RDAs, 10-11
Rebound effect and vitamin C, 153
Red blood cells, 4, 45, 79, 87, 92, 95,
124, 164-66, 174, 179, 221-22, 246
Reddened skin, 100
Reflexes, 81, 228
Renal dialysis, 263-64
Renal disease, 239, 243
Reproduction, 101-102, 163-64
Resorption, fetal, 247
Respiratory disease, 3
Restless legs syndrome, 82-86
Restlessness, 157
Reticulum cell sarcoma, 123
Retinitis, 275
Retinitis pigmentosa, 28
Retinol (vitamin A), 20
Retrolental fibroplasia, 175
Rheumatic fever, 25
Rheumatic heart disease, 170
Rheumatism, 68-69, 157
Riboflavin, 44-50
Rickets, 156-57, 229
Rocky Mountain Spotted Fever, 123
Rubella, 137
Rutin, 273

Sand, 251
Schizophrenia, 54-55, 70, 82-83, 146-
47, 210, 235, 265, 279
Schroeder, Dr. Henry, 205-206
Schwarz, Dr. Klaus, 269-70
Sciatica, 279
Scleroderma, 123, 178
Scoliosis, 157
Scurvy, 3, 127-28, 131-32, 138, 141,
150, 274
Seborrheic dermatitis, infantile, 102
Seizures, 228
Selenium, 235, 245-50, 257-58, 270
Senility, 83
Sepsis, 239
Serotonin, 71
Sexual function, 166-68, 258-59, 263-
64

Sexual maturation, 258
Sex vitamin, 163
Shute, Evan and Wilfred, 169–70
Sickle cell anemia, 89, 178–79, 262–63
Silicon, 251, 270
Silver, 249
Silver nitrate, 243
Sitophobia, 101
Skeleton, 190, 210, 238
Skin, 52–53, 57, 123–24, 126, 215, 228, 245, 252–53
Sleep, 52, 147
Sleepiness, 108
Small intestine, 93
Smell, sense of, 53, 258
Smoking, 150, 181–82
Sodium, 8, 255–56
   and magnesium, 228
   and potassium, 241–44
Sodium aminosalicylate, 98
Sodium ascorbate. *See* vitamin C
Sodium nitroprusside, 98
Soft water and heart disease, 196–97, 230
Spasms, 157, 228
Sperm, 166, 245
Spinal cord, 79–82, 107, 167
Spleen, 216
Spoon nails, 222
Steroid drugs, 148
Stiffness, 94
Stillbirths, 214
Stomatitis apthosa, 137
Stress, 14, 21, 24–25, 101, 105–110, 113, 127–28, 168, 202, 243, 259–60, 274
Stroke, 134, 170, 275
Stuttering, 40
Subclinical scurvy, 128
Sudden infant death syndrome, 40, 102–103, 228–29
Sugar and calcium, 199
Suicide, 95–96, 117
Sulfa drugs, 124, 185
Sulfisoxazole, 72
Sulfur, 269
Sunburn, 123
Sunlight and vitamin D, 155, 160
Sunscreen, 123
Supplements
   how to buy, 288
   necessity for, 12–13
Surgery, 111, 130–31, 210, 232, 243, 260–61

Sweat, 222, 243–44
Swelling, premenstrual, 69–70
Swimming and pantothenate, 109–10
"Synthetic" vitamin C, 154

Tannin, 42
Tardive dyskinesia, 75, 115–17, 235
Tartar, 179
Taste, sense of, 53, 209, 258
Tea and thiamine, 42
Teeth, 63, 126–27, 157, 190, 228, 238
   and fluoride, 213–17
Telangiectasia, 283
Tension
   and niacin, 53
   premenstrual, 69–70
Testicular degeneration, 247
Testosterone, 263–64
Tetanus, 38
Tetracycline, 151
Thalassemia, 179–80
Thallium, 249
Thiamine, 34–43
   and vitamin C, 149
Thirst, 216
Thrombin, 184
Thromboangiitis, 170
Thrombophlebitis, 169–70
Thrombosis, 177
Thymus gland, 126, 252, 258
Thyroid gland, 46, 101, 156, 216
Thyrotoxicosis, 219, 265
Thyroxin, 218
Tin, 270
Tingling, 68
"Tired blood," 221
Tiredness, 95–96, 108, 222
Titanium, 270
Tocopherol, 164
Tongue, 102
Toxic chemicals, 48, 74–75, 174
Tranquilizers, 50
Transcobalamines, 92
Trauma, 89, 232, 243, 274–75
Triglycerides, 132–34
Trimethoprim, 89
Tryptophan, 58, 60–62, 65, 67, 70, 77
Tuberculin test, 71
Tuberculosis, 74, 265
Tumors, 222
Typhus, 123

Ubiquinones, 245

Ulcers, 60, 77, 284
  cutaneous, 265
  intestinal, 110–11
  and niacin, 60
  pressure, 130
  and pyridoxine, 77
Ultraviolet light, 123
Uremia, 265
Urine formation, 237

Vanadium, 148, 270
Varicose veins, 276
Vascular disease, 255
Vasculitis, 178
Vegetarians, 77, 91, 110
  and cobalamin, 97–98
Visual purple, 20
Vision and thiamine, 38
Vitamin hysteria, 15–16
Vitamins
  defined, 6–7
  fat-soluble, defined, 15
  natural vs. synthetic, 288–90
  origin of term, 7
  vs. drugs, 286
  water-soluble, defined, 15
Vitamin A, 3, 19–33, 289–90
  and bioflavonoids, 275
  and vitamin C, 127
Vitamin B₁. *See* thiamine
Vitamin B₂. *See* riboflavin
Vitamin B₃. *See* niacin
Vitamin B₆. *See* pyridoxine
Vitamin B₁₂. *See* cobalamin
Vitamin B₁₅, 278–81
Vitamin B₁₇, 281–83
Vitamin C, 3, 125–54, 167, 289
  and adrenal cortex, 106–107
  and bioflavonoids, 273–76
  and cobalamin, 96, 98
  complex, 274
  and folate, 89–90

  and heart disease, 205
  and pantothenate, 106–107
  and riboflavin, 44
  and schizophrenia, 70
  and thiamine, 42
Vitamin D, 155–62, 289
  and calcium, 200
  and choline, 118
  and magnesium, 229
  natural and synthetic, 162
  and phosphorus, 238
Vitamin E, 163–83, 289
  cautions against use, 182
  natural and synthetic, 183
  and selenium, 246–48
  and vitamin A toxicity, 32
Vitamin K, 184–86
Vitamin P. *See* bioflavonoids
Vomiting, 267
  and potassium, 243

Water, 4
Weakness, 80–81, 94, 216, 222, 228, 244, 255
Weak pulse, 94
Weight loss, 235
Wernicke-Korsakoff Syndrome, 37
White blood cells, 136–37, 222, 246
Williams, Dr. Roger, 112, 151
Work and iron, 223

Xanthine oxidase, 84–85
Xerophthalmia, 23
Xerosis, 22

Zinc, 257–68
  and copper, 210
  and fiber, 290
  and folate, 89
  and schizophrenia, 70
  and vitamin C, 148